Medicine Hands

Therapists Workbook
and Journal

Medicine Hands

Therapists Workbook and Journal

Activities to Deepen Oncology Massage Practice

Gayle MacDonald, MS, LMT

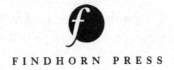

FINDHORN PRESS

Findhorn Press
One Park Street
Rochester, Vermont 05767
www.findhornpress.com

Findhorn Press is a division of Inner Traditions International

ISBN 978-1-84409-672-5

Cataloging-in-Publication Data for this title is available from the British Library

Printed and bound in the United States

Cover design by Richard Crookes
Text design and layout by Joan Pinkert
Reflections photograph by Ray Appel (zapple.ca)

IMPORTANT, PLEASE NOTE:
Prior to initiating the use of massage or any other touch
modalities, consult with the patient's doctor. *Medicine
Hands Therapists Workbook and Journal* is designed to be a
resource; it is not a substitute for medical advice. Different
state or municipal licensing boards have jurisdiction over the
practice of massage. These regulating bodies may have a policy
or recommendation with regard to massaging people with
cancer. Practitioners should become knowledgeable about
these regulations by contacting the licensing board.

May you be blessed to serve others.

*May you be blessed to do work that energizes your body,
fills your heart, and touches your soul.*

*May you blessed to see and feel your own beauty
through the work you do in the world.*

*May you be blessed to have people around you
that support your dreams and help them become a reality.*

ACKNOWLEDGEMENT
Three people in particular have supported me
to make this dream a reality:

Sharon Fisher, tech goddess, who brought the first draft to life;

Joan Pinkert, who went above and beyond the call of duty
in laying out the manuscript, advising and supporting;

Thierry Bogliolo, editor of Findhorn Press.

Contents

...in a bodywork session, I hold open the possibility that
people might become visible to themselves anew.
They may see and feel deeper thoughts,
bodily sensations and movements, emotions,
and sensing of spirit as if for the first time
or as if recalling a dream that actually immediately
seems more real than what had passed for reality.

—David Lauterstein, *Deep Massage Book*

The act of massage unites

heaven and earth,

spirit and matter,

divine and mundane.

—Gayle MacDonald,
Medicine Hands: Massage Therapy for People with Cancer

Preface

I coached a variety of sports in my former professional life—volleyball, basketball, swimming, and track and field. The thing that all sports have in common is the need for practice through repetition. Basketball players must do thousands of free throws and volleyball players thousands of serves; swimmers must put in an unfathomable number of laps in the pool; and runners, miles around the track.

In his book *Outliers,* Malcolm Gladwell presents research and interviews that address the relationship between hours of practice and achievement. According to Gladwell, it takes 10,000 hours to achieve mastery. Practice plays a major role in success, and there are no short cuts.

How does a massage therapist wanting to become adept at working with cancer patients accumulate practice? We study with teachers and on our own, participate in supervised hands-on practice, write case studies, get feedback from mentors, interact with peers, and give thousands of massages. *Medicine Hands Therapists Workbook and Journal* (MHTWJ) adds another aspect to the learning process. Through it, therapists are given a way to practice with the information in *Medicine Hands, 3rd Edition* so that it becomes more ingrained.

A workbook is the original self-paced learning system. Even though high-tech products are in vogue, I chose a slower, more proprioceptive way for the student to learn. Instincts told me that the kinesthetic process of recording answers and expressing feelings in writing, rather than by typing, would allow the reader to assimilate the information more thoroughly. As well, this style of learning is in alignment with the practice of massage for people living with cancer, which strives for the qualities of spaciousness and personal connection.

We are what we repeatedly do. Excellence, then, is not an act, but a habit.

—Aristotle

While I was writing MHTWJ, an article came to my attention that supported my instincts. The article was titled, "The Pen is Mightier Than the Keyboard," by Pam A. Mueller, Princeton University, and Daniel M Oppenheimer, UCLA. Mueller and Oppenheimer performed three different studies with their college students comparing the practice of taking notes on a laptop versus longhand. The two researchers found longhand note-taking to be more effective in the learning process. They found that "students who took notes on laptops performed worse on conceptual questions." The researchers surmised that this is due to shallower processing. Laptop note-takers tend to transcribe lectures verbatim rather than processing information and reframing it in their own words, as longhand note takers do.

The results of the above study didn't influence my decision to lay out the workbook/journal in print rather than in an electronic format. I was pleased, however, to find evidence for low-tech methods of learning.

Structure and Use

This workbook/journal is designed to be a supplemental learning source. It is best used in conjunction with guided lessons from an experienced teacher, hands-on experience, and interactions with peers. Some aspects of massage can be learned from webinars, online or distance-learning courses; however, live classwork with an experienced practitioner/teacher is required for other aspects.

The workbook/journal will appeal to the solo therapist concentrating on medically-oriented touch therapy; to student therapist groups studying oncology massage as part of their curriculum; to experienced therapists who want to review or deepen their practices; to teachers of cancer care massage; and to teachers within a general massage curriculum. It could also serve as a focal point for self-study, instructor-led class work, study groups that connect via email, a private Facebook page or other online group, Skype, or a monthly support group meeting.

The chapters of the workbook/journal correspond to the chapters in MH3. The only exception to this is Chapter 12, Caring for the Caregivers. It has been omitted.

Most chapters begin with a *Test Yourself* section, which emphasizes some of the main information from MH3. Following the Test Yourself feature are exercises that further enhance clinical knowledge, as well as nudge you to experiment with touch, words, and feelings. Below are some of these additional features:

- Pressure/Site/Positioning exercises.
- Case studies and massage planning.
- Awareness exercises.
- Reflective questions.
- Ethical dilemmas.
- Touch exercises.

Some readers may prefer to work sequentially through the chapters and their exercises, while others will choose to skip around, focusing on the material that most interests them. Either way will be effective.

MHTWJ makes a good traveling companion for train or plane trips or the commute to work. Reflection space exercises fit nicely on a plane trip or later at night when the house has quieted down. Many of the other exercises can be done when waiting for your child to finish swim team practice or orchestra. This workbook/journal may be something you do over a year's period of time, or longer.

Ample writing space is provided within the exercises for you to place handwritten answers. The only exceptions to this are the "Massage Session Planning" exercises in chapters 7, 8, 10, and 11. Readers will need to pause at these places, which are marked *Pause...and prepare*, to make photocopies of the needed forms. These can be found in the Appendices. An extra Reflection Space form is also included in the Appendices in case the spaces embedded in the text are insufficient in size.

On a practical level, users will want to have a 3-ring binder in which to place the Massage Session Planning worksheets. As well, I highly recommend laminating the cover or purchasing a plastic cover to protect it with.

Clues to the objective test features can be found by going to findhornpress.com/medhandsworkbook.

Personal Note

I hope this workbook and journal is useful in your studies. If you want to share an anecdote related to your use of it, I can be reached at: MedHands825@gmail.com.

Teachers, I am honored for this book to be used in your classrooms or with study groups. It was a labor of love and not created to be a source of great revenue. Findhorn Press set the price at a very economical level so that therapists and students can each afford to purchase a copy of their own. Because there are considerable costs associated with birthing a book, whether it is electronic or a printed copy, please honor the copyright and the work that such a book requires of the author as well as the publisher and do not reproduce it. Thank you.

Chapter 1

Introduction:
Cancer—A Part of Life

Chapter 1 of *Medicine Hands, 3rd Edition* (MH3) presented an overview of cancer from historical to modern times. It looked, too, at a future in which cancer continues its staggering effect on people worldwide due to aging, obesity and a host of other influences. Test yourself with the following questions as a way to review, highlight, and reinforce the reading from Chapter 1, and then we shall move on to new material.

Test Yourself

True-False: Place a T next to all true statements and an F next to those that are false. Correct all false statements and re-write them so that they are true. Most false statements can be corrected in more than one way.

Example: **F**   Cancer is an umbrella term for ~~ten~~ separate diseases. *hundreds of*

1. Part of the reason for an increase in cancer incidence is aging.

2. After smoking, parasite infections are the leading cause of cancer in the developed world.

3. Approximately 1 in 10 women in the US, UK and Australia have a chance of developing cancer in their lifetime.

4. The World Health Organization estimates that by 2050, the number of people older than 60 will triple, thus increasing the number of cancer cases.

5. The terms 'complementary' and 'alternative' can be used interchangeably.

6. Alternative therapies are defined as those that are used instead of or sometimes in conjunction with mainstream therapies to promote a cure.

7. Complementary therapies are used alongside conventional medicine, often to ease the side effects of the treatments.

8. Research has shown that massage can cure cancer.

9. Doctors and pharmacists are examples of ancillary or allied practitioners.

10. Massage therapists, physical therapists, and occupational therapists are examples of conventional practitioners.

11. An interdisciplinary care team might consist of doctors, nurses, pastoral care, a social worker, a massage therapist, an acupuncturist, nutritionist, and more.

12. Holistic care is a system that attends to the emotional and spiritual parts of a person.

13. Very few massage therapists will ever encounter people living with cancer.

Cancer—A Part of Life

Most people know someone affected by cancer. Even if you don't, you are affected by the vast numbers of people around you who are.

"Cancer." Notice your reaction to that word. Say it out loud to yourself or have someone else say it. Our presence and our touch can be affected by many variables, such as training, experience with family and friends, and beliefs. Without being aware of it, we can be affected by hearing certain terminology.

Becoming aware of our reactions to these words is important. Sometimes we pull away unconsciously when we hear a word. Literally, we pull away. But as touch therapists, we want to have the fullest contact possible. When we withdraw, even a little bit, we aren't fully present with the client. It is through the resolve to become more aware that we become conscious of where we hold steady with people and where we retract. Stop for a moment and examine your reaction to the words in the following exercises and then write about it in the space provided.

The hand that touches my body touches my life.

—Dianne Connelly, *Medicine Words*

Becoming Aware: The effect of words

Sit in a restful place, close your eyes, take a few breaths, rest for a few moments and then have someone read the following words, one at a time, with ample space in between each word (at least two minutes). Notice the responses that occur in your body. Is your breathing, the temperature of your body, or your sense of openness affected? Do you pull away or lean into the word? There are no correct responses, only awareness.

- Cancer
- Doctor
- Oncology
- Naturopath

Reflection Space

What did you notice about the effect each word had on you? In what way would your physical reaction to these words affect the quality of your presence or touch when massaging someone affected by cancer?

Cancer

Doctor

Oncology

Naturopath

Connecting with the Community of Practitioners

Health care is delivered by many types of care providers. Often times just *one* patient will be under the care of a long list of practitioners such as medical researchers, a variety of physicians including hospitalists, palliative care team, medical oncologists, radiation oncologists, and surgeons (e.g., oncology surgeon and cosmetic surgeon), scores of nurses, nurse practitioners, pharmacists, physician assistants, respiratory therapists, occupational therapists, physiotherapists, social workers, art therapists, and complementary therapy practitioners. By understanding more about these care providers, we as touch therapists can see the part we play in the total picture.

As well as being cared for by a multitude of medical, nursing, and ancillary practitioners, patients also create their own healing team that might consist of a support group, a physical therapist, massage practitioner, psychologist or yoga teacher. Understanding other types of therapists or clinicians and their roles in the patient's healing helps the practitioner engender respect for the type of support they can offer patients. This knowledge makes him or her a better team member, one who will be invited to work with the group of professionals who care for people with cancer.

Standards of Courtesy

The following section from the Society for Oncology Massage "Standards of Practice" gives excellent guidance in the matter of professionalism:

Conduct. The practitioner shall always behave in a professional and courteous manner when interacting with clients or medical professionals and encourage respect for all parties involved.

Professional Courtesy. The practitioner shall respect the qualifications or abilities of the physician(s) and other medical professionals. The practitioner shall interact with other professionals involved in the client's care to share information and provide for the best interest of the client while affirming the role of a massage practitioner as a member of the client's health care team.

Exercise 1:
Increase your understanding of other practitioners

The following exercise will help you become familiar with the education, licensing requirements, and type of care that various practitioners are trained to provide. Research this information using the various resources at your disposal, including qualified practitioners or the internet. (If you are doing these exercises with a partner, each of you could research four of the groupings and then report back to one other.)

	Education	Licensure requirement	Treatment goals
Art Therapist			
Licensed Clinical Social Worker			
Medical Oncologist			
Clinical Nurse Specialist in Oncology			
Music Therapist			
Naturopathic Physician			
Physical Therapist			
Yoga Instructor			

> ## *Build Your Practice:*
> ### Create a community resource list
>
> Create a resource list of allied specialists in cancer care for your clients. I vet other practitioners by asking questions about their training, by meeting or scheduling a session with them, and obtaining feedback from other practitioners or clients who are familiar with their work.
> - Yoga for people with cancer.
> - Exercise specialists (e.g., Lebed practitioners and personal fitness trainers).
> - Grief and support groups.
> - Meditation.
> - Counselors/social workers/psychologists/psychiatrists.
> - Cancer resource centers.
> - Acupuncturists, naturopaths and chiropractors who specialize in cancer care.
> - Lymphedema specialists.
> - Cancer retreat centers.
> - Spas (local and destination types) that offer care by trained therapists.
> - Aestheticians.
> - Website links (e.g., National Lymphedema Network, Macmillan Cancer Support).

Evaluating Websites

Other clinicians and practitioners are great resources, as is *Medicine Hands*. However, you will also need to use the internet as a main source of learning. Placed throughout MH3 are lists of websites. Let's explore and evaluate a group of lymphedema websites from around the world.

Pause...and prepare

A form, Evaluating Websites Worksheet, is provided on the page following the informational box. Make five photocopies, one for each website.

Exercise 2: Evaluating websites

Evaluate the following five websites using the five criteria listed in the informational box on the next page.
- Lymphoedema Support Network
  www.lymphoedema.org
- Lymphovenous Canada
  www.lymphovenous-canada.ca
- National Lymphedema Network
  www.lymphnet.org
- International Lymphoedema Framework
  www.lympho.org
- Reflexology Lymph Drainage
  www.reflexologylymphdrainage.co.uk

Criteria for evaluating a website

The internet is truly the people's forum, which is both an asset and a liability. It has connected us with people and information that would have been unimaginable 20 years ago. The rules governing it are minimal. Some sites have a managing editor; others are the work of a single person or a collaboration of people unaffiliated with large institutions. Verifying the credibility of web-based information is the responsibility of the reader. The following criteria will help when using the internet for research.

1. **Authority.** This reveals that the responsible person, institution or agency has the qualifications and knowledge to do so. When evaluating for authority, ask the following:
   a. Who is the author?
   b. Is the contact information clearly provided?
   c. What are the author's qualifications and professional background?
   d. Is the site is supported by an organization or a commercial entity?

2. **Purpose.** The intention of the information should be clear. Some sites are meant to inform, others to persuade or state an opinion, and some to entertain. Ask these questions when evaluating purpose:
   a. Does the content support the purpose of the site?
   b. Who is the target audience (students, academics, consumers, general readers)?
   c. Is the site organized and focused?
   d. Are the outside links appropriate for the site?

3. **Currency.** This area speaks to how up-to-date the website is. Look for this information:
   a. When was the content produced?
   b. How often is the site updated or maintained?
   c. Are the links up-to-date, reliable, and available?

4. **Objectivity.** Bias is another descriptor that could be used for this section. The content of all websites is partial in some way or another, which means it is impossible to measure objectivity. Information that resonates with the mainstream will be considered to be more objective. But truly, even material considered impartial is prejudiced in one way or another. The following questions will focus the reader's attention:
   a. What is the bias of this website?
   b. Is the site trying to explain, inform, persuade or sell something?
   c. Is there advertising that is in conflict with the content?

5. **Accuracy.** When trying to evaluate the veracity of the material, question the following:
   a. What is the author's affiliation?
   b. Does the information align with previous reading on the subject?
   c. Is the information comparable to other sites on the same topic?
   d. Does the text follow basic rules of grammar, spelling, and composition?
   e. Is a bibliography or reference list included?

(Adapted from Dalhousie University website. Available at: http://libraries.dal.ca/using the library/evaluating web resources/6 criteria for websites.html accessed April 3, 2015.)

Evaluating Websites Worksheet

1. **Authority.** Does the responsible person, institution or agency have the qualifications and knowledge to do this?

2. **Purpose.** The intention of the information should be clear. Is it meant to inform, persuade, state an opinion, or entertain?

3. **Currency.** How up-to-date is the website?

4. **Objectivity.** How partial or impartial is the material?

5. **Accuracy.** Evaluate the truthfulness of the material.

Ethics Dilemma

Below is a common dilemma of post-graduate massage practitioners:

"The massage school I attended gives massage in the school clinic to people with cancer, however, the only instruction we were given as students was to work gently with these clients. Should I speak to the clinic director about the need for more education?"

Reflection Space

List three dilemmas central to this situation. Here's #1 to get you started:

1. What is the school's liability when it doesn't provide adequate training to students working with people with cancer?

2.

3.

Final Thoughts

The cancer incidence rate will not lessen in the near future. It will be "all hands on deck"—oncologists, nurses, naturopaths, acupuncturists, social workers, massage therapists, and more—to provide the needed care. My dream is that healthcare gravitates more and more toward interdisciplinary teams and that massage therapists attain a level of skill and acceptance that enables them to work alongside other providers as team members. As a discipline, oncology massage has a long way to go to develop the expertise to sit around the table when patient care meetings are called. In 20 years I've learned a lot. Lately I've seen how much I, and we, don't know. It is such a paradox: the longer you live, the more you realize what you don't know.

Chapter 2

Understanding Cancer and Metastasis:
Biology, Not Mechanics

Chapter 2 in MH3 describes metastasis as simply as possible. However, understanding the rudiments of it is still very complicated. In this chapter, no new material will be introduced. The focus will be on mastering the basics of what was presented in the text.

Becoming Adept with Language

To become adept at using the language of a profession, practice is required. The following exercises push you to learn the definitions of words and gives practice utilizing them.

Exercise 1: Flash cards

Make flash cards of the following words with the definition or description on the back.

- Acquired mutations
- Angiogenesis
- Apoptosis
- Carcinogen
- Carcinoma
- Cell surface receptors
- Cytokines
- Dysplasia

- Epigenetics
- Epithelium
- Grading
- Growth factors
- Hematological cancers
- Hyperplasia
- Hypoxia
- In situ

- Inflammatory process
- Inherited mutations
- Metaplasia
- Metastases
- Metastasis
- Neovascularization
- Sarcoma
- Staging

Becoming Aware: **The effect of words on touch**

Sit in a restful place, close your eyes, take a few breaths, rest for a few moments and then have someone read the following words, one at a time, with ample space in between each word (at least two minutes). Notice the responses that occur in your body. Is your breathing, the temperature of your body, or your sense of openness affected? Do you pull away or lean into the word? There are no correct responses, only awareness.

- Mutation
- Metastasis
- Contraindicated
- Stage

Reflection Space

Record what you have noticed about each word in the space provided. Would your reaction to these words affect the quality of your presence or touch when massaging someone affected by cancer?

Mutation
Metastasis
Contraindicated
Stage

Test Yourself: **Matching**

Draw a line from the word in the left-hand column to the correct definition on the right.

Carcinomas	Cancers that affect the blood, bone marrow, and lymphatic tissue.
In situ	Cancers that arise from bone, muscle, connective tissue.
Sarcomas	Programmed cell death.
Apoptosis	Cancers that begin in epithelial cells.
Hyperplasia	Cancer still contained in the boundaries of the original tissue.
Hematological	Precancerous growth pattern.

Exercise 2: **Creating a sentence**

Use the following words in a sentence that shows understanding of the term.

Example: **Epithelium**   *Epithelium lines the GI tract.*

Carcinoma	
Hematology	
Inherited	
Metastases	
Chromosome	
Interstitium	
In situ	
Dysplasia	
Carcinogen	

Exercise 3: **Make a list**

List five carcinogens that can lead to acquired mutations.

1.	
2.	
3.	
4.	
5.	

Perhaps you listed viruses as possible carcinogens. List three viruses that have connections with the rise of cancer. Next to the virus, list the type of cancer associated with it.

Virus	Type of cancer
1.	
2.	
3.	

BR CA 1 and 2 are the two most commonly known inherited genes. List three other inherited mutations and the kinds of cancers they lead to.

Inherited mutation	Type of cancer
1.	
2.	
3.	

List five qualities possessed by cancer cells (MH3, pages 20-21).

1.	
2.	
3.	
4.	
5.	

List five factors that influence the development of cancer in individuals (MH3, pages 22-23).

1.	
2.	
3.	
4.	
5.	

After examining the process of metastasis, list the four implications for bodywork (MH3, page 23).

1.	
2.	
3.	
4.	

Exercise 4: **Short answer**

In your own words, summarize the process by which damage can occur to the DNA (described on page 14 of MH3).

Briefly describe the relationship between inflammation and cancer (MH3, page 16).

Test Yourself

True-False: Place a T next to all true statements and an F next to those that are false. Correct all false statements and re-write them so that they are true. Most false statements can be corrected in more than one way.

Examples:

F   ~~Leukemia~~ is an example of a carcinoma.   *Breast cancer*

F   Leukemia is an example of a ~~carcinoma~~.   *hematological cancer*

Generic questions

1. Cancer is an umbrella term that covers many different diseases.

2. The majority of tumors occur in epithelial tissue.

3. The majority of cancers are hematological in nature.

4. A tumor is defined as cancerous if it has the ability to be invasive.

5. Grading is the process of determining how advanced a cancer is.

Genetics questions

1. The majority of genetic mutations are inherited.

2. BR CA 1 is an example of an acquired genetic mutation.

3. Too much sun exposure can cause acquired mutations.

4. Some viruses can cause cells to mutate, which contributes to the cancer potential.

5. Epithelial cells are at higher risk for mutations because they are constantly replicating themselves. Each time a cell divides, there is a risk of error.

Epigenetics questions

1. Epigenetics is the study of changes in gene expression caused by reasons other than alterations in the DNA sequence.

2. Once epigenetic damage has occurred, it is permanent.

3. Epigenetic modifications do not change the DNA sequence, they affect how cells read the genes.

4. Cell surface receptors act like antennae, reading the contents of the interstitial fluid.

5. The interstitial fluid contains elements such as chromosomes and inherited mutations.

Fill-in: Use the words below to fill in the following sentences:

- **inside**   - **cell surface receptors**   - **epigenetics**

- **chromosomes**   - **nucleus**   - **blood**   - **lymphatic**

1. The genetic material that provides the body's blueprint is contained on _____.

2. The reproductive control center of the cell is the _____.

3. The majority of mutations have their beginnings in highly active cells such as epithelium,

_____, and _____.

4. DNA delivers messages to the cell from the _____.

5. Outside messages to cells are delivered via _____.

6. These outside messages make up the study of _____.

Final Thoughts

Recently one of our massage interns was sharing a story about a new client with stage 4 metastatic breast cancer in the lungs and hip. The therapist explained to the woman what her planned course of action would be, that it wouldn't be deep massage, and the reason why. In order to explain the rationale behind the massage adjustments, the therapist must have some basic understanding of what is occurring in the deeper layers of a client's body due to the disease and the treatments. Attaining this knowledge requires intentional, focused study of how cancer starts and spreads.

Chapter 3

Touch—Rx for Body, Mind, and Heart:
A Review of the Research

Research literacy is a vast topic that can be given only limited attention in a single chapter. The aim in these few pages will be to attend to some basic, but nonetheless important, research knowledge as well as to increase your level of discernment. Let's start by rating your comfort level with the topic of research. We will repeat the same scale at the end of the chapter as a post-test.

Becoming Aware: **Comfort level with research**

> **Pre-test**
> Using a Likert Scale, indicate how comfortable you are right now with the topic of 'research' by circling the number that corresponds to your comfort level.
>
> | 1 | 2 | 3 | 4 | 5 |
> |---|---|---|---|---|
> | uncomfortable | | | | comfortable |

Exercise 1: **Flash cards**

Make flash cards of the following words with the definition or description on the back.

- Anecdotal evidence
- Case study
- Convenience sample
- Control group
- Crossover design
- Experimental group
- Feasibility study
- Hypothesis

- Intervention
- Meta-analysis
- Methodology
- Outcome measure
- Placebo effect
- Pre- to post-test design
- Qualitative research
- Quantitative research

- Randomized controlled trial
- Retrospective study
- Scientific evidence
- Statistical significance
- Trend
- Variable

Before we begin on other exercises, test yourself on the material in MH3.

Test Yourself: **Research basics**

Fill-in: Use the following words to complete the sentences below. Each word should be used only once.

- anecdotal
- qualitative
- standard
- respiratory rate
- control
- meta-analysis
- statistical significance
- trend
- blood pressure
- quantitative
- randomized
- heart rate

1. A client who reports sleeping better the night of a massage is giving
_____ evidence.

2. A study that splits the group of subjects arbitrarily into two groups is referred to as
_____.

3. A randomized controlled study always has at least one experimental group and one
_____ group.

4. A study that collects heart rate and blood pressure before the massage, 15 minutes after, and 60 minutes after is a _____ study.

5. A _____ shows a certain direction but is not statistically significant.

6. The control group in a study is the one that receives the _____ intervention.

7. If you performed a study that interviewed three people who have received touch therapies alongside their cancer treatment, asking them each the same three questions, this would be considered _____ research.

8. Analysis that proves the results are not due to chance or error: _____

9. _____ is a method of examining a group of studies that meet certain criteria.

10. List the three vital signs often used in research to monitor a person's response to the experimental intervention:
a._____   b. _____   c. _____

True-False: What the evidence shows.
Place a T next to all true statements and an F next to those that are false.
Correct all false statements and re-write them so that they are true. Most
false statements can be corrected in more than one way.
Example:
F   ~~The scientific research~~ shows that constipation can improve from a
reflexology treatment.   *Anecdotal evidence*

1. Massage often relieves pain and anxiety in the short term.

2. The scientific evidence shows conclusive results between nausea relief and massage.

3. The symptom that patients report as being most problematic is fatigue.

4. The effects of massage on immune function are well studied.

5. Only a handful of studies have been performed on massage and the sleep of people with cancer. The findings are inconclusive.

6. The research shows that hospital stays are shortened when patients receive massage during their stay.

7. Depression clearly shows statistically significant improvement from the use of touch therapies.

8. Occasionally, individuals can decrease the use of pain medications, but on the whole, the research doesn't support the notion that the use of massage will lead to less pain medication use.

9. The scientific evidence shows that heart and breathing rates consistently decrease as a result of touch therapies.

10. Cancer patients often report improved sleep as a result of massage, however, there are too few studies to form a concrete conclusion.

Aspects of Research

Some practitioners want to be able read the original research article, which is the best way to truly understand the details. However, it takes a fair amount of effort and education to become facile at this. The average therapist is happy enough to get their research information from second- or third-hand reviews of the original paper, such as those that appear in massage publications, on the internet or the nightly news. The goal in this limited space is to focus on the needs of the average therapist, to help them become more discerning about research reports and their sources.

There are a number of aspects to research. For this chapter we are going to focus on four:

- Finding research—the basics
- General questions to ask yourself
- Discerning the levels of evidence
- Analysis of the abstract portion of the research study

Finding Research

> ### *Research Tools*
> Vetted scales on sleep, quality of life, pain, and neuropathy can be found at the IN-CAM Outcomes Database: http://www. incamresearch.ca/glossary

The person keen to find original research will use resources such as university libraries, medical and nursing journals, and/or the Cochrane Collaboration database. However, for our down-to-earth approach, there are some easier ways to access research using the internet. Sometimes the general public is allowed full entry to the original research article via the internet. At other times only the abstract can be accessed for free, while the full text must be purchased.

- Explore academic search engines, such as:
  - *Google Scholar:* www.ScholarGoogle.com
  - *Web Lens:* www.weblens.org/scholar.html
  - *Educational Technology and Mobile Learning:* www.educatorstechnology.com/2013/02/ 12-fabulous-academic-search-engines.html

- Search the www.Pubmed.com or the www.Biomedcentral.com websites. Enter key phrases such as "cancer and complementary therapies," "breast cancer and massage therapy research," or "massage and constipation research."

- You will find many oncology massage research studies listed at these two resources:
  - *www.tracywalton.com*
  - Reference section at the end of Chapter 3 in *Medicine Hands, 3rd. Ed.*

General Questions to Ask

All research adds to the total picture regarding the benefits of massage. There are layers of questions to ask when assessing which research is strongest. When surveying original research projects, the following questions give some sense as to the weight of the research.

In what journal was the article published?
Different journals have different standings. *Massage and Bodywork* has much less gravitas than the *Journal of Pain Management. Oncology Nursing Forum* carries way more influence than *Prevention Magazine.* The research reports contained in massage journals carry less weight than what is found in research or oncology journals. Massage magazines do not carry original research. But thank goodness for having someone who interprets the research for us. It is a time-consuming activity to read original research!

In what year was the article published?
Older CAM studies tend not to be as rigorous. Newer studies have the advantage of being able to build upon what has come before them.

What is the background or experience of the investigators?
Serious research projects must have a primary investigator, usually someone who has a doctoral degree. Then you will notice the other investigators may be RNs, PTs and statisticians. The massage therapists are generally listed last because they are the ones who carry out the massage but don't design the study, gather or analyze the data.

Was the study funded? If so, by whom?
For instance, a study funded by Johnson and Johnson has a lesser weight than one funded by the National Cancer Institute.

Exercise 1: Comparing abstracts

Using PubMed, read the abstracts or full articles from the following four studies. Rate them by placing an "S" if they are strong or a "W" if they are weak, according to the criteria listed above. You may need to dig a bit deeper to find the background of the investigators. (Hint: Use your favorite research engine, such as Google, Bing, Duckduckgo.)

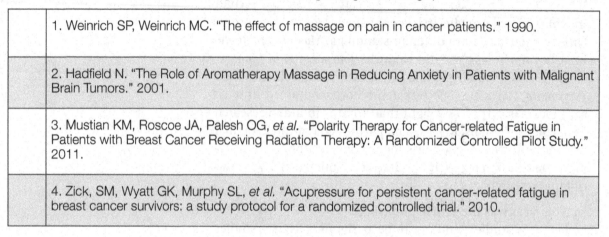

	1. Weinrich SP, Weinrich MC. "The effect of massage on pain in cancer patients." 1990.
	2. Hadfield N. "The Role of Aromatherapy Massage in Reducing Anxiety in Patients with Malignant Brain Tumors." 2001.
	3. Mustian KM, Roscoe JA, Palesh OG, *et al*. "Polarity Therapy for Cancer-related Fatigue in Patients with Breast Cancer Receiving Radiation Therapy: A Randomized Controlled Pilot Study." 2011.
	4. Zick, SM, Wyatt GK, Murphy SL, *et al*. "Acupressure for persistent cancer-related fatigue in breast cancer survivors: a study protocol for a randomized controlled trial." 2010.

Discerning Levels of Evidence

Some studies carry more weight than others because of the type of study or how they were designed. A variety of factors give weight to a study—the sample size, the use of a control group, randomization, the level of statistical analysis, and the qualifications of the researchers, to name some.

Exercise 2: Types of evidence

Below are five types of evidence listed in a random order. Using your basic understanding of research from MH3, arrange the levels of evidence. Place a 1 next to the evidence you would consider the strongest, proceeding to a 5 for the weakest.

	Case report
	Randomized, controlled trial
	Anecdote
	Meta-analysis
	Pre- to post-treatment, no control

Not only do certain types of evidence hold more weight, so, too, do certain resources. Some websites are for the purpose of information only and are created by very weighty organizations, such as the National Health Service (UK) or the National Institutes for Health (US). Other websites that include research are trying to market something, which always gives it less gravitas because it is biased toward a product. Usually, research is reported second- or third-hand and there is no way to know the expertise or bias of the reporter, which dilutes the information compared to the original article.

Exercise 3: **Rank these resources**

Place a 1 next to the resource you would consider the strongest proceeding to a 5 for the weakest.

	Massage journal
	Pubmed—www.pubmed.gov (National Institutes of Health—U.S.)
	General search engine, such as Google, Bing, or Duckduckgo
	Beauty or health magazine
	Peer-reviewed nursing journal

Analyzing the Abstract

An abstract is the first section within an original piece of research or case study. It is an overview. While important information is lost by not reading the entire article, a reading of the abstract gives the therapist an adequate amount of basic information. Below is a screen shot of an abstract.

Auton Neurosci. 2009 Oct 5;150(1-2):111-5. doi: 10.1016/j.autneu.2009.03.010. Epub 2009 Apr 18.

The effect of massage on immune function and stress in women with breast cancer--a randomized controlled trial.

Billhult A[1], Lindholm C, Gunnarsson R, Stener-Victorin E.

⊕ Author information

Abstract

OBJECTIVES: To examine the short-term effects of light pressure effleurage on circulating lymphocytes by studying the number and activity of peripheral blood natural killer (NK) cells in patients with breast cancer compared to a control group. Furthermore, the effect of light pressure effleurage on salivary cortisol levels, heart rate and blood pressure was studied.

DESIGN: Single centre, prospective, randomized and controlled study.

METHODS: Thirty women, aged 50 to 75 years (mean 61 sd=7.2) with breast cancer undergoing radiation therapy in a hospital in southwestern Sweden were enrolled in the study. They were allocated to either receive massage in the form of a full-body light pressure effleurage treatment, or a control visit where they were given an equal amount of attention. Blood samples, saliva, notation of heart rate and blood pressure were collected before and after massage/control visit. Differences in change over time between groups were analyzed by Student's t-test.

RESULTS: Light pressure effleurage massage decreased the deterioration of NK cell activity occurring during radiation therapy. Furthermore it lowered heart rate and systolic blood pressure. No effects were demonstrated on cortisol and diastolic pressure.

CONCLUSIONS: A single full-body light pressure effleurage massage has a short-term effect on NK cell activity, systolic blood pressure and heart rate in patients with breast cancer. However, the long-term clinical importance of these findings needs to be further investigated.

PMID: 19376750 [PubMed - indexed for MEDLINE]

An abstract should contain the following:
1. A precise statement of the research question.
2. A description of the design.
3. Information about the subjects.
4. The main outcome measures.
5. The results.
6. Researchers' conclusions.

The above abstract is very complete in its presentation. Let's analyze the abstract on the following page using the same criterion. Not all abstracts are created equally.

Int J Neurosci. 2005 Apr;115(4):495-510.

Natural killer cells and lymphocytes increase in women with breast cancer following massage therapy.

Hernandez-Reif M[1], Field T, Ironson G, Beutler J, Vera Y, Hurley J, Fletcher MA, Schanberg S, Kuhn C, Fraser M.

⊕ Author information

Abstract

Women diagnosed with breast cancer received massage therapy or practiced progressive muscle relaxation (PMR) for 30-min sessions 3 times a week for 5 weeks or received standard treatment. The massage therapy and relaxation groups reported less depressed mood, anxiety, and pain immediately after their first and last sessions. By the end of the study, however, only the massage therapy group reported being less depressed and less angry and having more vigor. Dopamine levels, Natural Killer cells, and lymphocytes also increased from the first to the last day of the study for the massage therapy group. These findings highlight the benefit of these complementary therapies, most particularly massage therapy, for women with breast cancer.

PMID: 15809216 [PubMed - indexed for MEDLINE]

Exercise 4: Analyzing an abstract

Comment on the strengths or weaknesses of each part of the abstract from Hernandez-Reif, *et al.*

1.	A precise statement of the research question.
2.	A description of the design.
3.	Information about the subjects.
4.	The main outcome measures.
5.	The results.
6.	Researchers' conclusions.

Becoming Aware: **Comfort level with research**

Post-test
Using a Likert Scale, indicate how comfortable you are right now with the topic of 'research' by circling the number that corresponds to your comfort level.

1	2	3	4	5
uncomfortable				comfortable

Reflection Space

From the pre- to the post-test, did your Likert Scale score change? List three ways in which you feel more comfortable with the topic of research.

By performing the pre- and post-test in this chapter, you have participated in research of a sort. You have measured your own comfort level with the topic of research topic prior to the start of an intervention and following the intervention. In this case, the intervention was the presentation of education material and exercises. We could turn this into a research study. Our research question would be: Does reading about massage basics and participating in written exercises affect the confidence of massage therapists in the area of research basics?

Build Your Practice: **Research in private practice**

- Create a Research Corner either on your website, a bulletin board or in a newsletter. Download links to abstracts or research reviews.
- Collect simple data from your consistent clients regarding one or two variables, such as energy or pain. Ask them before and after each session to rate the variable using a 1 to 5 Likert scale. Over time, surveying this information might show helpful trends.

Final Thoughts

Reading original research requires a certain mindset and does not appeal to many practitioners. The purpose of this chapter is to allow those who don't want to specialize in research to put their toes into the research waters, so to speak, just to become a little more comfortable. Therapists wishing to develop more expertise should seek out Martha Menard's book, *Making Sense of Research* and *Massage Therapy: Integrating Research and Practice*, edited by Trish Dryden and Christopher Moyer.

Trish Dryden, a Canadian researcher, said something I've never forgotten: "No evidence doesn't mean it doesn't work." This surely applies to massage in cancer care. Few outcomes have received adequate study, thus there is no evidence one way or the other about its effectiveness on a group of people.

Our one level of evidence in many cases is the individual anecdote, which is powerful, to be sure. However, touch practitioners need to accurately represent the evidence. If our proof is anecdotal, we need to depict it as such. When there is sufficient scientific research, such as with short-term pain and anxiety, we can share that. Most often, though, there are either only a few studies, or the research is inconclusive, or there is not yet any research. That is what we must convey.

Chapter 4

The Side Effects of Cancer Treatment:
Why the Need for a Less Demanding Approach

Chapter 4 lays the foundation for the next six chapters. An understanding of the side effects caused by cancer treatments informs every part of the massage session. At this point we are not yet applying this information to the massage, we are only trying to have a better understanding of the treatments.

Exercise 1: **Flash cards**

Make flash cards of the following words found in Chapter 4 of MH3. Place the definition or description on the back.

- Absolute neutrophil count
- Amygdala
- Analgesic
- Anticoagulant
- Antineoplastic
- Brachytherapy
- Coagulation
- Diuretic

- Emetic
- Erythropoiesis
- Hematopoietic
- Hippocampus
- Immunotherapies
- Limbic system
- Myelosuppression
- Narcotics

- Neutropenia
- Neutrophils
- Osteonecrosis
- Palliative
- PTSD
- Thrombocytopenia
- Trauma
- Venuous thromboembolism

Surgery

Surgery is often performed in the pursuit of a cure or to reduce the size of the tumor prior to chemotherapy or radiation. It may also be part of palliative action to make the person more comfortable. Surgery is sometimes used to prevent a dire problem, such as a blockage, or it may be used for cosmetic reasons.

Exercise 2: **Short- and long-term effects of surgery**

Place an X in the appropriate box that indicates whether the symptom is primarily a short- or long-term side effect of surgery. Short-term, in this exercise, is defined as a few months. Beyond that is considered long-term. Sometimes it can be both short- and long-term.

	Short-term	Long-term
Risk of lymphedema from nodal dissection		
Constipation		
Fatigue		
Adhesions		
Risk of blood clot development		
Body image issues		
Numbness or hypersensitivity adjacent to surgical site		
Depression of the immune system		
Swelling and inflammation at incisional site		
Discomfort from surgical positioning		
Unconscious guarding of the surgical or procedural site		

Test Yourself: Surgery

True-False: Place a T next to all true statements and an F next to those that are false. Correct all false statements and re-write them so that they are true. Most false statements can be corrected in more than one way.

1. It wasn't until the 20th century that small, localized cancers could be cured with the use of surgery.

2. Surgery and radiation were the main forms of cancer treatment until the 1960s.

3. Surgery is always performed before radiation therapy.

4. Following surgery, a person could have gentle touch therapy as soon as they are back in their hospital room.

5. Surgery stimulates a surge of platelets to staunch the flow of blood at the surgical site.

6. Following surgery, the body is repairing blood and lymphatic vessels damaged from the incision.

7. Digestion and elimination speed up following surgery.

8. A surgical patient is at less risk for the development of blood clots.

9. Positioning on the surgical table is responsible for a great deal of muscular discomfort.

10. Lymph nodes are commonly removed to investigate the stage of the cancer. This procedure puts people at risk for lipedema.

Radiation

Radiotherapy, for the most part, is a localized treatment. It is used to eliminate the disease, shrink the tumor prior to surgery, or to improve a patient's quality of life by controlling symptoms. The two following exercises will help you to understand the side effects of the most commonly used type of radiation, external beam radiation.

Exercise 3:
Side effects of radiotherapy for neck and throat cancer

Mr. H received external beam radiotherapy for tonsil cancer. The field of treatment included the mouth out to the cervical lymph nodes behind the ears, the jaw, throat, SCM, and all of the tissue down to the supraclavicular region. The side effects from this treatment are based on the anatomical areas in the field of treatment.

Think about the anatomical features that exist in this area, such as teeth, taste buds, thyroid and many more. Bear in mind that the radiotherapy beam affects the tissue along the pathway, exiting on the opposite side. List five possible side effects that Mr. H might experience and the reason for each.

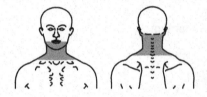

Example:
Dry mouth due to damage to the salivary glands

1.	
2.	
3.	
4.	
5.	

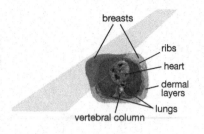

breasts
ribs
heart
dermal layers
lungs
vertebral column

Exercise 4:
Side effects of radiation therapy for breast cancer

Ms. S was treated for breast cancer on the left side. The treatment was delivered at multiple angles. In this exercise, the goal is to follow the pathway of just one of the angles and think through the anatomical areas that might be affected. Underline the anatomical structures below that would be affected by this radiation beam:

Left side subcutaneous layer (anterior and lateral)

Left side epidermal and dermal layers (anterior and lateral chest wall)

Left side ribs

Right lung

Sternum

Heart

Kidneys

Stomach

Left side internal and external intercostal muscles

Left maxilla

Fascial layers (anterior and lateral chest wall)

Left Ilium

Left side pectoralis

Test Yourself: Radiation

True-False: Place a T next to all true statements and an F next to those that are false. Correct all false statements and re-write them so that they are true. Most false statements can be corrected in more than one way.

1. External beam radiation causes the molecular bonds in cells to break, which ultimately causes the cell contents to spill into adjacent areas.

2. Bone in the field of radiation therapy treatment develops fragility within the first month after treatment ends.

3. Brachytherapy is another name for external beam radiotherapy.

4. The most common way to deliver radiation is internally.

5. People receiving external beam radiation are not radioactive.

Multiple choice: Mark all of the correct choices. There may be more than one correct answer.

1. Which of the following are common short-term side effects of radiotherapy?

   a. Increase in white blood cells

   b. Bleeding ulcers

   c. Fatigue

   d. Skin issues in the field of treatment

2. Which of the following are common long-term side effects of external beam radiotherapy?

   a. Secondary cancers

   b. Tendons and other connective tissue may be less pliable in the field of treatment

   c. Low blood counts

   d. Radioactivity

3. One of the main causes of tissue damage from external beam radiation is:

   a. Decreased white blood cells

   b. Fatigue

   c. Inflammation

   d. Edema

4. Bones can become fragile because of:

 a. Certain chemotherapies

 b. External beam radiotherapy

 c. Certain hormone changes

 d. Bone metastases

5. People treated with radiation for colorectal, gynecological, or prostate cancer might experience which of the following side effects?

 a. Hair loss

 b. Incontinence

 c. Sexual dysfunction

 d. Shortness of breath

6. The medical term for bone marrow suppression is:

 a. Pancytosuppression

 b. Immunosuppression

 c. Myelosuppression

 d. Suppression gravitas

Chemotherapy

Antineoplastic agents are given for many reasons: to reduce the
size of large, bulky tumors before surgery; to increase the sensitivity of the cancer to other therapy, such as radiation; to treat
cancers that can metastasize; or to treat tumors that may not have
spread but are, for some reason, inoperable or in locations where
radiation is inadvisable.

Exercise 5: Short answer

Antineoplastic agents, commonly referred to as chemotherapy, are designed
to kill the tumor cells. Describe what happens physiologically when the cells
are killed.

There are three common side effects from bone marrow suppression.
What are they?

1.	
2.	
3.	

People are at greater risk of blood clots when receiving chemotherapy.
List three reasons why.

1.

2.

3.

List the names of three different chemotherapies that put patients at greater
risk of blood clot development. Place the generic name first, followed by the
trade name.
Example: *carboplatin (Paraplatin)*

1.

2.

3.

Test Yourself: **Chemotherapy**

True-False: Place a T next to all true statements and an F next to those that are false. Correct all false statements and re-write them so that they are true. Most false statements can be corrected in more than one way.

1. Often, two or more chemotherapies are used in order to damage cancer cells at different stages in the cell division process.

2. When cells are killed, the contents leak out and generally go into the circulatory system.

3. Cytokines are an example of biochemical released from cells' content, which can cause inflammation, fever, and tissue destruction.

4. The absolute neutrophil count is one indication of how quickly blood coagulates.

5. One of the common side effects of hematopoietic growth factors, such as pegfilgrastim (Neulasta), is deep bone pain.

6. Biotherapies, also referred to as immunotherapies, cause fairly mild reactions in the body.

7. Many antineoplastic drugs suppress bone marrow production.

8. Some anticancer medications cause long-term side effects to organs, joints, and cognition.

Test Yourself: **Matching**

Draw a line from the word in the left-hand column to the correct definition on the right.

Analgesic	Used to prevent blood clots from forming or to assist in dissolving blood clots.
Anticoagulant	Drugs that increase urine output.
Antiemetic	A group of drugs that work by stimulating the immune system.
Biotherapies	Drugs used to control nausea and vomiting.
Diuretic	Pain relief medication.

Pause...

We've been focused on the cognitive learning pieces so far in this chapter. Brain work! Let's pause for a moment in the midst of this review about surgery, radiation, and chemotherapy and notice another part of our being: our emotions. It can be sobering to learn about these forms of treatment. We have emotional responses to them, which should be recognized. For instance, I often notice how quiet the room becomes when I am talking about radiation. It affects the listener on every level. Space needs to be made for the emotional response. Holistic learning includes not only the mind, but also the heart and body.

Reflection Space

What have you noticed emotionally as you re-read the material in this chapter of MH3? Did your body reflect your feelings in any way, such as by breathing or postural changes? Did the material empower you or disturb you? Were you surprised by anything that you read?

Emotional Demands of Cancer

While we are in a reflective mode, let's continue from that place and think back to the information presented in MH3 about the emotional demands of cancer, including trauma. Traumas are caused by a variety of events and are unique to each individual. I experience mild symptoms of it when I go to the dentist, while on the other hand, a friend of mine loves going to the dentist. Compassion for and understanding of each other's distress can be developed by examining our own. Trauma may seem to be an emotional event, but it also has a physiological component. The body carries a story that is often overlooked.

Reflection Space

Look back at the "Symptoms of trauma" listed on page 91 in MH3. Reflect on one thing that can distress you, such as having an injection, being on a cramped bus, or having an area massaged that you are protective of. How do you respond physically and emotionally? Does your heart beat fast or your head swim? Is your breathing affected? Do you have an urge to do something such as curl up, run, or fight?

Exercise 6: **Short answer**

Knowledge of the limbic system will help in understanding your own and others' emotional reactions. The limbic system is composed of two parts, the hippocampus and the amygdala. In your own words, describe each of them. Study of the amygdala in particular helps to understand the phenomenon of being re-traumatized.

Hippocampus
Amygdala

Test Yourself: **Emotional demands of cancer**

True-False: Place a T next to all true statements and an F next to those that are false. Correct all false statements and re-write them so that they are true. Most false statements can be corrected in more than one way.

1. The emotional demands of the cancer experience can be experienced as threat or danger and thus stimulate the parasympathetic nervous system.

2. Trauma re-wires the brain and changes its chemistry.

3. The limbic system can't always distinguish between a traumatic occurrence and an event that is meant to be helpful.

4. Elements of a massage session can inadvertently trigger trauma.

5. Difficulty with coherent thinking can occur when the sympathetic nervous system is triggered.

Fill-in: Use these words to fill in the following sentences:

- **sympathetic**   - **digestion**   - **dilate**   - **constrict**
- **gentler**   - **safety**   - **touch**   - **breathing**

1. In order to shift the nervous system into the restful, parasympathetic branch, massage strokes must be slower and _____.

2. Deep bodywork stimulates the_____ nervous system.

3. Unconscious coping mechanisms occur in order to create a sense of_____.

4. When people feel unsafe, the fight or flight response can cause the heart and _____ to accelerate, _____ slows or stops. Blood vessels _____ in muscles and _____ in other parts of the body.

5. Warm blankets, special objects, and _____ are just some of the ways to create a sense of safety when clients are feeling extremely vulnerable.

Final Thoughts

At the risk of being repetitious, I want to re-emphasize: Devote time to learning about the treatments. Once you understand them, the massage adjustments will come naturally. This is not to exclude the study of the actual disease and its side effects, but it is the treatments that will require the majority of massage adjustments.

Pressure, Site, and Position:
An Organizational Framework

Planning a touch therapy session is made simpler by using the pressure, site, and position categories. In the following pages, we will practice applying this organizational framework to a variety of situations. Based on your reading of Chapter 5 in MH3, let's warm up with the exercise below. It asks you to list the main adjustments needed for ten common side effects.

Test Yourself

Pressure, Site or Position? Below the following side effects, list the primary adjustment that is called for: Pressure, Site, or Position. While you might be able to list all three of the categories, there is one *primary* answer.

1. Fatigue	6. Peripheral neuropathy
2. Easy bruising or bleeding	7. New incision
3. Bone metastases	8. Area of herpes outbreak
4. Neutropenic fever	9. Pain medication
5. Medical device	10. Shortness of breath

Adjusting for Cancer Treatment

The three main forms of cancer treatment are surgery, chemotherapy and radiation. Exercises 1 through 3 give you practice in categorizing the needed adjustments for each form of treatment using pressure, site, and positioning. For now, the exercises are simplified to only include the side effects caused by each particular form of treatment rather than an accumulation of side effects.

Exercise 1: Side effects from a surgery

Following surgery, a person could have a gentle foot massage, in most cases, as soon as they return to their hospital room. Once they are allowed to have a fuller session, the pressure/site/position format can be used to think through the needed adjustments. The following patient had his right kidney removed. The variables from his situation are listed below.

Place an X in the boxes that correspond with each adjustment. Some side effects may require two or three adjustments. If the condition calls for reduced pressure, also record in the box whether the pressure should be a 'systemic' reduction or a 'local' one. For instance, peripheral neuropathy is a localized pressure precaution to the feet whereas thrombocytopenia calls for a systemic, generalized reduction in pressure.

	Pressure *Systemic or Local?*	Site	Position
Example: 1. Incision R flank	X Local	X	X
2. Incisional pain			
3. Pain medication			
4. Fatigue			
5. Blood clot risk			

Exercise 2: Side effects of cyclophosphamide

Let's use the pressure/site/position framework to categorize the side effects from a single chemotherapy that is common in patients' drug regimens: cyclophosphamide (Cytoxan). Some of the side effects of this chemotherapy are listed below. Place an X in the box(es) that corresponds with the adjustments needed for each side effect. Some conditions may require two or three adjustments. Indicate whether pressure precautions are systemic or local.

In this exercise, only one medication has been used. Normally, a patient in treatment for cancer will be on five to ten medications, including chemotherapies. Even those in recovery may still be on a number of drugs for a variety of conditions, such as depression or pain.

	Pressure *Systemic or Local?*	Site	Position
1. Fatigue			
2. Nausea and vomiting			
3. Hair loss			
4. Neutropenia			
5. Neutropenic fever			
6. Thrombocytopenia			
7. Risk of blood clots			
8. Edema in feet and lower legs			
9. Joint pain			
10. Increased uric acid			
11. Lower back or side pain (related to kidney disease)			

Exercise 3: **Side effects from radiation**

Now that you are warmed up, let's look at two different time periods for someone being treated for breast cancer with radiation. Part A of the exercise lists the side effects as she is going through radiotherapy. Part B fast-forwards five years. For simplification, only her radiation side effects are listed here; this client might have others related to surgery or chemotherapy.

A. Side effects during treatment

	Pressure *Systemic or Local?*	Site	Position
1. Fatigue			
2. Severe skin tenderness in field of treatment			
3. Reduced ROM shoulder on treated side			
4. Shingles outbreak under treated breast			
5. Pain medication for shingles			

B. Side effects five years later

	Pressure *Systemic or Local?*	Site	Position
1. Reduced ROM of shoulder on treated side			
2. Slight swelling in upper arm			
3. Fibrotic tissue in the chest			
4. Radiation–induced osteoporosis in thoracic vertebrae and ribs			

Pressure Exercises

The next three exercises deal in one way or another with the pressure of massage strokes. This is the most-often needed adjustment for people in treatment and recovery as well as those who are many years out from treatment.

Instructions — "COLOR Me Pressure Guidelines"

Gather together five crayons or colored pencils (not gel pens) that closely resemble the colors of peach, plum, tangerine, lime, and brown. These are the hues used for the Pressure Guidelines in MH3, page 101. Color in the "COLOR Me" chart on the next page using hues that correlate to those on page 101. Not only do the colors need to match, but so too does the depth of color. Make note how light the saturation is on the peach color (pressure 1). The saturation of the plum color is a bit more (pressure number 2), and so on with the tangerine and lime colors. Notice what changes you make in the use of your pencil or crayon in order to match the depth of color. Your pressure will probably change as well as other things.

(**Alternative version:** If you don't have colored implements available, a leaded pencil can be used for the exercise. Rather than matching the colors from MH3, page 101, use the pencil to match the gray shade used to highlight each of the numbers of the "COLOR Me" chart on the next page.)

COLOR Me Pressure Guidelines

0/1	Off the body or Light touch	• Energy technique or light touch • Skin contact • Nurturing • Slow • Full hand • As if contacting a ripe PEACH	Severe side effects:	– Blood clot – Bone mets or osteoporosis – Bruising – Edema – End of life – Fatigue – Fever – Fragile – Nausea – Neuropathy – Trauma
2	Superficial muscle	• Contact with superficial muscle • Nurturing • Slow • Full hand • As if gently and slowly washing a PLUM	Moderate side effects:	– Bone mets or osteoporosis – Bruising risk – Fatigue – In-treatment – LE risk – Neuropathy – Trauma
3	Slightly firm	• Slightly firm muscle contact • Inch forward • Not forceful • Not ambitious • As if massaging a TANGERINE	Improving side effects:	– Increased energy – Ready to find "new normal" – Significantly recovered from Tx
4	Firm controlled	• Firm, controlled pressure • Goal-oriented • As if squeezing a LIME	Full recovery:	– 100% recovered – Excellent bone / tissue health – No LE risk – Physically fit
5	Heavy, forceful	Heavy, forceful pressure is rarely appropriate for those who have been through cancer treatment. Most people who have experienced treatment will have some residual side effects and are not candidates for heavy, forceful massage pressure.		

Reflection Space

What did you notice about the application of greater and greater pressure with the crayon or pencil? Did you notice other factors as you shaded in the increasingly deeper colors? Is there any correlation in your experience to this exercise and massage?

Try This: **Touch exercise**

While massaging a partner, experiment with your hands in the following positions while giving long, gliding strokes. Both giver and receiver should remain mindful of what they are noticing from each of the variations. When deep pressure can't be used, the fullness of hand contact is very important, as you will see from this exercise.

- Slightly tented in a shallow A-shape.
- Finger pads only.
- Thumb up.
- Little finger up.
- Full-handed contact with the fingers touching together.
  (When using full-handed contact, every part of the hand and fingers are in contact with the partner's tissue.)
- Full-handed contact with the fingers relaxed apart.

Reflection Space

What did each of you notice during this experiment? Did you have preferences? Did one hand position feel more confident, or less? Was there a greater sense of presence from one position over another?

Ethics Dilemma

A colleague who is trained to massage people with cancer posed the following situation to me:

> "A friend and I receive massage from the same therapist. My friend has a history of breast cancer treatment and still has peripheral neuropathy and is at risk for lymphedema. This massage therapist works very deeply on me. Often I feel like I was run over by a truck for a couple of days following the massage. I am wondering how to ask my friend what kind of pressure our mutual massage therapist uses on her? Should I ask the practitioner, who is also in my professional orbit, if she is adjusting correctly for my friend? What are the ethics around this?"

Reflection Space

There is no one way to approach this scenario. List three possibilities for this situation that would not cross professional boundaries with either the therapist or the friend.

Positioning Exercises

The following three exercises ask you to notice or experiment with positioning—both the client's and the therapist's.

Exercise 4: Positioning of the therapist

Examine the body mechanics of the therapists below. List two things that all of these therapists are doing to ensure their own physical comfort, which then translates through their hands to the client as comfort.

1.	
2.	

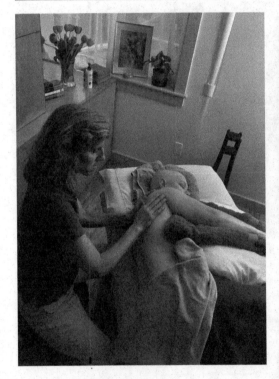

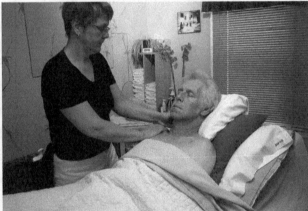

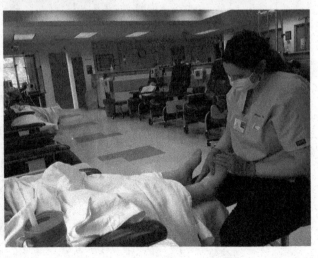

Left photo by Nanci Newton
Courtesy of Tracy Walton and Associates

Upper right photo by Elvira Yanez

Lower right photo by Gayle MacDonald

Exercise 5: **Positioning of clients**

What one thing could each therapist in these photos do to increase the patient's comfort? You will find clues in the previous photos. Record your answers in the space below.

1.	
2.	
3.	

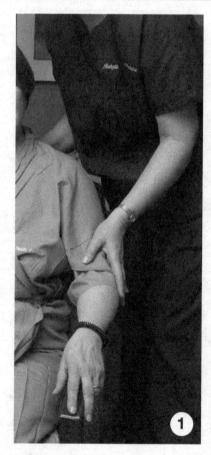

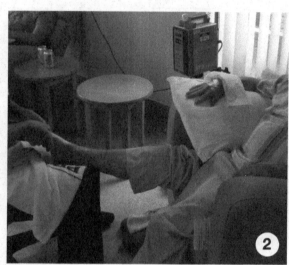

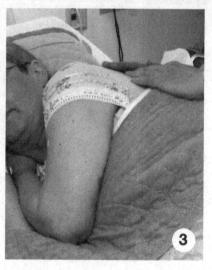

Left photo by David J. Lawton

Upper right photo by Maggi Scott

Lower right photo by David J. Lawton

Try This:
Creating more comfort on the massage table

With a partner, experiment with the following ways that might increase a client's comfort. You may not personally like them all, but even those of you who have been in practice for years will find techniques that you might not have guessed would provide so much more relaxation on the table.

- In supine position, try a pillow under the knees instead of a bolster. Which do you prefer?
- Have your partner place something under your heels as well. Some people prefer a towel, some a flat pillow, and others like a pillow that is similar in size to the knee pillow. Really, just try it! See which you prefer. Most people, once they've experimented with it, will find that their back is more relaxed with something under the heels.
- When prone, ask your partner to place a hand towel under your shoulders. Clients who've had breast surgery may feel more comfortable with this support, as may people with shoulder issues.
- When prone, experiment with a folded bath towel under your midriff or farther down toward the hips.

Reflection Space

Did anything from these experiments surprise you? Did you discover new ways to be comfortable on the massage table or to help your partner be more fully relaxed with the use of positioning?

Final Thoughts

The goal of the pressure/site/position framework is simplicity. It allows the therapist to gather up a great deal of information and channel it into a few different categories. We could distill the process down even further to one basic question: "How can the massage session be made less demanding?" That is the deeper goal within each category, finding ways to adjust the level of demand so that is appropriate to each person's situation.

Besides moderating the pressure, taking care around specific sites of the body, and exploring positioning until the ultimate comfort is found, there are a handful of other variables that help to lessen the demand of a massage session. The length of the session can be shortened; vigorous modalities can be swapped out for gentler ones; less abrasive skin products can be substituted; or the volume of the music can be adjusted. How you position pillows, enter and move around the massage room, or bring your hands to rest on the client's body—all can be adjusted to be less demanding.

In Chapter 6, the focus will be on the process of gathering information. Once again, pressure, site, and positioning categories will have a place in the scheme of things.

Chapter 6

Gathering Information:
An Essential Part of the
Massage Session

Massage therapists, by and large, feel a variety of stresses about the gathering of health information from clients, such as time, client reticence, and lack of knowledge. Becoming skilled at this part of the session takes practice, experience, and dedication to the importance of the consultation process. In this chapter we will practice with some communication concepts that are familiar but may have not been given enough attention for you to feel skillful with them.

Let's warm up by testing yourself on what you read in Chapter 6 of MH3.

Test Yourself

True-False: Place a T next to all true statements and an F next to those that are false. Correct all false statements and re-write them so that they are true. Most false statements can be corrected in more than one way.

1. Start the intake process with the question, "Is there anything I need to know?"

2. There are a few instances when it is OK to not consult with the client about their health.

3. The therapist has the primary responsibility for gathering the health information needed for a safe massage.

4. Nurses know what information to give a massage therapist regarding a client or patient's health.

5. Clients receiving care in outpatient settings can have foot massage without the therapist gathering any health information.

Open-ended/Closed-ended: Place an "O" next to the questions that are open-ended and a "C" next to those that are closed-ended. Re-write the closed-ended questions so that they are open-ended. (*Example:* If I asked a client, "is the music OK?" it is a closed-ended question. To make it open-ended, I could ask, "What kinds of music do you like for massage?")

1. Tell me about your chemotherapy treatment.

2. Is this pressure OK?

3. Would it be OK if I massage your abdomen?

4. What are you noticing about this area of your body?

5. Is this almond oil OK?

Client-centered/Therapist-centered: Place a "C" next to the questions/statements that are client-centered and a "T" next to the ones that are therapist-centered. Re-write the therapist-centered questions so that they are client-centered. (*Example*: The question, "Would it be OK if I massage your incision?" is very therapist-centered. It can be made client-centered by saying, "Shall we include the incision in the massage session, or leave it out?")

1. Would you like me to massage your feet?

2. Would it be OK if I massage your head?

3. Tell me which areas you would like massaged.

4. I usually start people face down, is that OK?

5. Are there areas of your body that you protect?

Holistic Communication

Linear communication is quick and straightforward. It employs tick boxes, organizes information via body systems, and uses closed-ended questions that lead to "yes," "no," and "fine." Most of us have a great deal of experience with this way of gathering information from clients.

Holistic communication attends not only to words, but to the breath, to eyes that open wide or eyes that scrutinize, to fingers or feet that are restless or still. It hears the long pause, gives credence to a tone change, and listens to facial expression, because often, the truth is not in the words. Becoming sensitive to these forms of expression requires time and commitment.

Exercise 1: Just listen

With a partner, sit across from one another and each take a turn answering this prompt, "Tell me about your morning." Each person is to talk for five minutes. It doesn't sound like long, but it can be when you aren't used to silence. The job of the listener is only to listen. Don't give any feedback or ask any questions. Just listen and be aware—notice the speaker's hesitations, eyes, face, restlessness or stillness, and all the other ways your partner is communicating nonverbally. Notice when their voice softens or becomes energized, be aware of silences, detours, breaths and hesitations.

While you are being mindful of your partner's expressions, notice your inner reactions. As you listen, notice how your face and body express themselves. Are you really listening? Or are you half listening and half forming a reply in your head as your partner talks? The goal of this exercise is to put all of your attention on the speaker, to listen with minimal insertion of yourself.

As we went through the referral form she said it was so nice for someone to spend so much time asking her these questions and really listening to what she had to say. She felt that once she had finished her chemo no one wanted to ask about her burnt skin, etc. Each person was only interested in their part, not looking at her as a whole and all the things that were still affecting her since her treatments.

—Jacqueline George, LMT, Pittsburgh, PA

Reflection Space

What was it like to listen and be listened to without interruption? What was easy, what was hard? What surprised you? What was the quality of your listening? In what other ways besides words did your partner communicate to you?

Gathering Information

In live classes, we spend time practicing how to obtain open-ended feedback. I challenge the participants to NOT use the question, "Is that OK?" for an entire weekend. It's difficult! By the end of three days, some progress is made, but when therapists return home they lapse back into the old routines. The new habit is not yet well-grooved.

In this section, let's try to re-pattern our questioning strategies in three different parts of a massage session: the intake process, during the session, and afterwards.

Try This: Questions that promote stories

Try including some open-ended questions like those below when gathering a person's health history. They promote stories rather than ticks in a box.

Instructions: Use a highlighter to underscore one or two questions that you would like to practice for a week. The questions can be used with all clients, not just those who are medically complex.

- How would you like massage to support you?

- What is the healthiest thing about your body?

- What does your body need in order to heal?

- What would it mean to live well?

- What brings you comfort?

- What is standing between you and peace in this moment?

- What's your understanding of what is happening?

- Are there areas you protect?

- Tell me about your scars. Old and new.

- Are you prone to swelling anywhere?

I had a guest whose energy was high from the moment I picked her up in the lounge. She kept talking over me and giving me quick "No" answers when I first began my usual intake. She rambled on and on and was clearly trying to disrobe to get on the table before I was done speaking. I stopped talking, took a brief silent deep inhale and held eye contact with her. In a gentle, calm voice, I asked if she had any areas that she might be protective of?

For whatever reason that one specific question made her stop still, she thought a bit and then calmly said "Yes, my head." There was no elaboration, but from that moment on, her energy had shifted and her whole being relaxed. It's as if my initial standard questions were just cookie cutter to her and not important. But that one specific question and how it was asked made her feel like I suddenly connected in a way that allowed her to feel comfortable enough to just be in my presence without the nervous energy of chatter.

—Sharon, Phoenix, AZ

Reflection Space

Which question(s) did you choose? What responses did you get from clients or practice partners? Did this questioning strategy shift anything for you or your client? Did you notice any carry-over into other areas of your life from practicing "story" questions?

Try This: *Replace "Is that OK?"*

The question, "Is that OK?" often leads to "Yes." or "Fine." Sometimes it is a useful query, but often by asking for feedback in more open ways, you can discover helpful particulars that will improve the session. How else can you inquire about such things as pressure, comfort, or areas to be massaged? Return to page 113 in MH3 for reminders. Be sure that your questions are client-centered. Try this for a week, or even a day.

Reflection Space

Describe one or two of the questions you substituted for, "Is that OK?" What was it like for you to try to delete that question from your repertoire for a day? How did your clients respond?

Try This: **Follow up within 48 hours**

If you wait until the client's next session to ask for feedback, they will most likely have forgotten it by then. Contacting them within 48 hours will help the client become aware of how the massage affected them, and it will allow you to obtain specific feedback. When asking for follow-up feedback, there are two important qualities to the questions: are they specific and are they open-ended? By asking specific questions, we obtain valuable information about the effects of the massage. Open-ended questions create an invitation for people to share honestly rather than be led to the answers that we, as therapists, may want.

Part 1: Feedback questions
Instructions: Which of the following questions meet the above two qualifications of being specific and open-ended? Place a check mark next to them.

	1. I am calling to see how you are.
	2. Tell me about your sleep last night.
	3. I am hoping you felt better after yesterday's massage.
	4. I am calling to be sure you don't have any soreness after the massage.
	5. What has your energy been like since the massage?
	6. Did you sleep better?
	7. What did you notice about your appetite?
	8. Did you feel more relaxed?

Part 2: Follow-up practice

For the next week, do one follow-up a day with a chosen client. The contact can be made via phone, email, or text. It will be helpful at first to write out your questions ahead of time. In the following space, list two basic questions that you would like to ask everyone. I always ask these two questions:

Tell me about your energy since the massage.

What has your sleep been like?

List your own questions below. (Feel free to use the same ones I use.)

1.	
2.	

Reflection Space

What did you like about contacting clients within 48 hours? Was there anything you disliked?

Ethics Dilemma

A hospital massage therapist wrote seeking advice for the following situation.

"A friend who lives on my street is also a patient at the hospital where I work, and I've been very involved with her care. She was recently admitted to the hospital again, this time, with a very poor prognosis. I can't go anywhere in my neighborhood without being asked whether I think she is coming home. I'm feeling very stressed with this repeated question. I've responded that I don't know, but it feels like a lie. Can you give me some help with a better response?"

Reflection Space

One suggested answer that I gave to this therapist was, "Because I work at the hospital, I can't give information about patients. But I could give you the hospital address and you could send her a card so she knows you are thinking about her." We all have had times where we didn't know what to say in situations like this or we said too much. Reflect about a time when this happened to you and how you would handle it now in hindsight.

Communicating with Health Care Professionals

There is no sure-fire recipe for success in communicating with health care professionals. Some therapists make contact using an introductory letter delivered in person. (Sending material without human contact almost never elicits a response.) Others find success when one professional refers the therapist to colleagues. Besides doctors, other professionals who are supportive of massage therapy are social workers, psychotherapists, nurses, physiatrists, physical and occupational therapists, acupuncturists, naturopaths, and chiropractors. Therapists have shared that giving rack cards or business cards to other professionals can be helpful in making people aware of their services.

Suggestions for communicating with professionals

- Keep the correspondence brief and factual.
- Do not send anything that takes more than a glance to understand
- Speak their language.
- Have documents copyedited to insure that the presentation of letters and promotional materials are professional in every way.

Suggestions for creating promotional materials

- Allow spaciousness between sections. Too much on a page is overwhelming.
- Present the benefits accurately. If scientific research is inconclusive, cite the benefit as anecdotal evidence.
- Use real photos, preferably of yourself massaging real clients rather stock photos.

Build Your Practice: Creating a resource packet

A business practice must be built brick by brick. Even therapists hired as hospital employees or within a wellness center must 'sell' their service and build a clientele, not unlike a private practitioner. Every time I approach a patient in their hospital room, in the waiting area, or in their chemo chair to see if they would like a massage, I am gently promoting, educating, and sharing what I have to offer. Massage, in the eyes of patients and other healthcare providers, is not an essential service in the way nursing or respiratory care is.

A resource packet can be created to educate patients and professionals. The contents need to be specific to the audience, environment, and patient group. Following are some content examples:

- **A short letter to the patient's health care provider** that lists the adjustments you will be making for the client. (See Appendix 1, Sample Letter to Health Care Provider.)

- **Promotional material and business card.**

- **Articles:** The following articles are available on the internet at no charge. It can be difficult for massage therapists without a hospital affiliation to garner many of the articles available due to high fees charged by professional journals. When gathering articles for the packet of a professional, insert articles published in professional journals rather than magazines, such as *Prevention Magazine, Massage Magazine,* or a local news article. Articles from magazines are more appropriate for client packets. Copies of the following articles could be placed in a professional packet.

  - Corbin L. Safety and efficacy of massage therapy of patients with cancer. *Cancer Control.* 2005 Jul;12(3):158-64. Available at: http://www.ncbi.nlm.nih.gov/pubmed/16062163

  - Cassileth BR, Vickers AJ. Massage therapy for symptom control: outcome study at a major cancer center. *Journal of Pain and Symptom Management.* 2004;28(3):244–249. Available at: http://www.jpsmjournal.com/article/S0885-3924(04)00262-3/fulltext

  - Zick SM, Alrawi S, Merel G., *et al.* Relaxation Acupressure Reduces Persistent Cancer-Related Fatigue Epub 2010. Available at: http://www.ncbi.nlm.nih.gov/pmc/articles/PMC2949582/

- **A list of potential benefits of massage for the person affected by cancer.** See Appendix 2: Sample List of Potential Benefits of Massage for People with Cancer in the back of the book for a list of potential benefits. Please notice the use of the word 'potential.' Scientific research is only clear about the effects of massage on two variables: short-term pain and short-term anxiety. Other benefits have not been researched to any certainty. They are supported mainly by anecdotal evidence.

Final Thoughts

We all have many ingrained practices that we perform unconsciously. Some of this is an outcome of our conditioning and other behaviors are because of training. Old patterns, such as the question, "Is that OK?" are difficult to change. Moving toward new expressions of communication, such as open-ended questions, requires a huge commitment, usually a year of concerted effort. And yet, the payoff is worth the work. It makes a more spacious place for our clients to connect with themselves.

Chapter 7

First Do No Harm:
Adjusting for the Common Side Effects of Cancer Treatment

The directive to "First Do No Harm" is a guiding principle, originally for physicians, that no matter what treatment is being delivered, the patient's well-being is the primary consideration. In order to accomplish this, one of the things a therapist must become adept at is dealing with the information shared by medically complex clients. Part of this capability requires memorization of medical terms, a few lab values, and clinical considerations. Let's see how you are doing with this facet.

Exercise 1: Flash cards

Before "Testing Yourself," make flash cards of a few new words that were used in Chapter 7 of MH3.

- Alopecia
- Co-morbidity
- Edema

- Graft v. host disease (GVHD)
- Hand-foot syndrome

- Hypercoagulation
- Intrathecal

Test Yourself

Multiple choice: Mark all of the correct choices. There may be more than one correct answer.

1. Which three of the following side effects have the potential to cause severe harm to a client?

   a. An absolute neutrophil count of less than 1,000

   b. Chronic alopecia

   c. A platelet count of less than 20,000

   d. Venous thromboembolic (blood clot) disorders

2. Constipation can be caused by which of the following?

   a. Narcotic pain medications

   b. Dehydration

   c. Low platelets

   d. Chemotherapy

3. Chemotherapy-induced peripheral neuropathy can cause:

   a. Pain or numbness

   b. Redness of the skin

   c. Adhesions to the connective tissue

   d. Damage to sensory nerves

4. Neutropenia can develop because of:

a. Low electrolytes

b. Bone marrow suppression due to chemotherapy

c. Leukemia

d. Fatigue

True-False: Place a T next to all true statements and an F next to those that are false. Correct all false statements and re-write them so that they are true. Most false statements can be corrected in more than one way.

1. A person with shingles may be contagious until the last blister has scabbed over.

2. The main adjustment for chemotherapy-induced peripheral neuropathy is positioning.

3. Fatigue from cancer treatment is usually resolved within six months.

4. Hand-foot syndrome is similar to chemotherapy-induced peripheral neuropathy (CIPN).

5. If adjusted, touch therapy can be given to a post-op patient within hours of the surgery.

6. Smoking is an example of a co-morbidity.

7. Someone with a platelet count between 20,000 and 50,000 can safely receive a firm pressure massage.

8. Central IV catheters can cause the development of a blood clot in the area.

Fill-in

1. The medical term for low platelets is _____.

2. The medical term for a low white blood cell count is _____.

3. The accumulation of fluid in the peritoneal cavity is referred to as _____.

4. The prime adjustment for fatigue is _____.

5. The normal range for platelets is _____.

6. List three reasons people in cancer treatment might experience pain:
_____, _____, and _____.

7. List three contributing factors to the creation of edema in people receiving cancer treatment:
_____, _____, and _____.

8. List three factors that can contribute to fatigue: _____,
_____, and _____.

Planning the Massage Session

Initially, it is cumbersome to gather and translate information that is new to us. Our flow is disrupted, we feel awkward and unskilled. Learning to play a musical instrument or strike a volleyball is much the same. In order to become fluid, tasks must be broken down into various steps and then practiced, practiced, practiced. Eventually, with much repetition, the separate pieces come together into oneness. This takes time and practice.

Working with people in treatment is less about fixing and more about "being with." The majority of people who are in treatment will benefit most from a level 1 or 2 pressure. Occasionally, level 3 is appropriate for select people.

Below is the part of the Pressure Guidelines from MH3, page 101, and reproduced in Chapter 5 of this workbook that is most commonly applied to people in treatment. When planning a massage session for someone in treatment, the following influences will most often be in play. There is not one aspect that is clearly more important than another. All three must be taken into account in shaping the session.

- The desires of the client.
- The training and background of the therapist.
- Side effects of cancer treatment and other health factors.

0/1	Off the body or Light touch	• Energy technique or light touch • Skin contact • Nurturing • Slow • Full hand • As if contacting a ripe PEACH	Severe side effects:	– Blood clot – Bone mets or osteoporosis – Bruising – Edema – End of life – Fatigue – Fever – Fragile – Nausea – Neuropathy – Trauma
2	Superficial muscle	• Contact with superficial muscle • Nurturing • Slow • Full hand • As if gently and slowly washing a PLUM	Moderate side effects:	– Bone mets or osteoporosis – Bruising risk – Fatigue – In-treatment – LE risk – Neuropathy – Trauma

No matter whether a client is currently in treatment or many years out, the pressure/site/position framework is the centerpiece around which the massage plan is formed. It requires massaging many hundreds of clients to develop ease with organizing the clinical information in your mind. So, let's practice a bit.

In the Appendices section, Appendix 3, Massage Session Planning Worksheet, is set up around the pressure/site/position framework. Another form, Appendix 4, Medications Worksheet, has been created to help you consolidate your research of client medications. These forms will also be used with clients referred to in chapters 7, 8, 10, and 11.

Pause...and prepare

Make a photocopy of each:

- **Appendix 3, Massage Session Planning Worksheet**
- **Appendix 4, Medications Worksheet**

First, let's look at samples that use these two forms with Client A. Her medical history can be found within Appendix 5a. Following this are Appendix 5b, the Medications Worksheet and Appendix 5c, the Massage Session Planning Worksheet for Client A. These two samples will give you an idea of how to proceed with Clients B and C, which are found below in Exercises 1 and 2.

Exercise 1: *Planning the massage session—Client B*

As you read the medical history of Client B:

1. Summarize her cancer treatment history at the top of the **Massage Session Planning Worksheet**.

2. List her *possible* pressure, site and positioning needs.

3. List Client B's drugs and chemotherapies on the **Medications Worksheet**. Using reliable resources, list the reason for taking each drug and its common side effects.

4. Is there any information from the **Medications Worksheet** that might be relevant to planning the massage session? If so, list it on the **Massage Session Planning Worksheet**.

Client B

Medical History:

Client B is a 64-year-old woman diagnosed with stage 4 ovarian cancer. She was having low back pain and went to the doctor secondary to the pain not going away. Ovarian cancer with metastases in the lining of her lungs was found, and chemo treatments were started to decrease the size of the tumor prior to a hysterectomy. She was given a chemo regimen of six cycles of taxol and carboplatin every three weeks. Six weeks following the end of chemo, a complete hysterectomy was performed. Eight inguinal lymph nodes were removed bilaterally. This was two months ago. B is very quiet and reserved and seems to be very depressed.

Medications *(past and current):*

(past)

- Taxol
- carboplatin
- Xanax

(current)

- Neurontin
- morphine sulfate
- Effexor

Side effects of treatment and disease:

- **Fatigue**—a result of the chemo treatments and also a residue from the surgery.
- **Nausea**—a residue of chemotherapy and current medications.
- **Peripheral neuropathy**—a result of chemotherapy.
- **Joint pain**—a residual of the Taxol.
- **Anxiety**—a result of diagnosis of cancer, fear of the future, and shortness of breath.
- **Shortness of breath**—a result of the lung metastases.
- **Insomnia**—due to hormonal changes, anxiety, pain.
- **Loss of hair**—due to chemotherapy.

Pause...and prepare

Make a photocopy of each:

- **Appendix 3, Massage Session Planning Worksheet**
- **Appendix 4, Medications Worksheet**

Exercise 2: **Planning the massage session—Client C**

Now let's use the same framework with a more complex person, Client C. Repeat the process undertaken with in Exercise 1 with Client B.

Client C

Medical History:

Client C is a 61-year-old man with stage 4 metastatic colon cancer to the lungs. He was originally diagnosed with stage 3 colon cancer four years ago. The following month he had a colon resection but did not need a colostomy bag. The month following that he started a 6-month treatment plan of six treatments of Folfox and six treatments of oxaliplatin. He suffers from severe neuropathy in his feet due to the chemotherapy. A month after that, three months post-diagnosis, Client C had a pulmonary embolism and was prescribed Coumadin, which he is still on. At the end of chemotherapy, his scans showed no evidence of cancer.

Three and a half years after the discovery of the initial colon cancer he was diagnosed with stage 4 metastatic colon cancer in his lungs and immediately began Fluoroucil (5 FU) and Camptosar. He received this treatment every other week for 12 months. Three months ago this regimen was stopped. At that time, his scans showed that the lung nodules were shrinking. Client C is now on maintenance chemotherapy, 5 FU and Avastin, every other week.

In addition to the colon cancer, he suffers from hypothyroidism and anxiety.

Medications (past and current):

(past)

- Coumadin
- 5FU
- Avastin
- Camptosar (3 mos. ago)
- Ativan

(current)

- Zoloft
- Ambien
- Synthroid
- Prilosec
- Vitamin D-3
- Neurontin

Side effects of treatment and disease:

- **Thrombocytopenia**—due to 5FU. At the lowest, platelets were 60,000.
- **Neutropenia**—due to 5FU. Presently, neutrophil count is 1,500.
- **Neuropathy**—due to the first round of chemotherapy drugs four years ago (Folfox and oxaliplatin).
- **Diarrhea**—due to chemotherapy (5FU) and Zoloft.
- **Fatigue**—as a result of the chemotherapy. He is not working, so the lack of social interaction keeps him closed up at home and contributes to his fatigue.
- **Insomnia**—particularly severe after his chemo treatments.
- **Shortness of breath**—a result of the lung tumors; however, this only affects him if he does extreme exertion.
- **Low back pain**—due to chemotherapy but also due to the fact that Client C is overweight and inactive (poor core strength).

Test Yourself

Let's test your clinical thinking skills and your ability to put together the whole picture. Client C is fatigued due to chemotherapy, but there are additional conditions besides chemotherapy that might be contributing to this.

Fill-in: List as many influences as you can in the space below. (I count 9 at least.)

1.

2.

3.

4.

5.

6.

7.

8.

9.

Try This: *Ultra-careful v. full-hand contact*

Often when preparing to massage a client in treatment, such as clients B and C, I hear therapists express that they are going to be "ultra-careful" when they touch the client. This changes the way they touch a person. I can feel the therapist drawing away from the client before they've even met. Of course I want therapists to take care, but fear-based care is not satisfying to anyone. Try the experiment below and see how the words you use when talking to yourself affects your touch and presence.

With a partner:

1. Hold the phrase 'ultra-careful' in your mind as you massage for a minute or two. Stop and ask for your partner's feedback.

2. Hold the phrase 'full-handed contact' in your mind as you massage for another minute or two. How does that affect your touch, your posture, and your mindset?

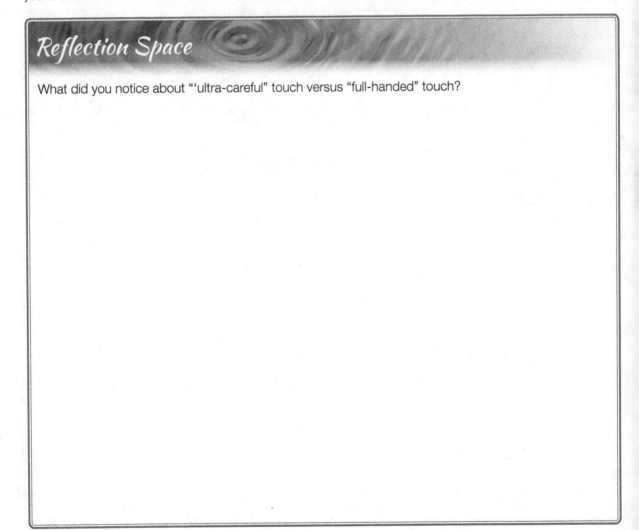

Reflection Space

What did you notice about "'ultra-careful" touch versus "full-handed" touch?

Becoming Aware: **The effect of words**

Our identity as massage therapists is often at odds with the adjustments needed by clients in treatment for cancer. A shift in how we define ourselves is frequently needed in order to become the practitioner a medically complex person requires. Claiming a new title is often all it takes. Sit in a restful place, close your eyes, take a few breaths, rest for a moment and then try on several identities and notice how each affects you physically. Allow ample space between each.

- Massage therapist
- Touch therapist
- Complementary Therapist

Reflection Space

Record the sensations you felt in your body with each identity.

Massage therapist

Touch therapist

Complementary therapist

Ethics Dilemma

People with cancer, or who are being treated for it, ask for deep pressure as often as any other clients. Even people in the hospital with desperately low platelets or with bone pain from Neulasta request firm pressure. They believe that deep, uncompromising pressure is the answer to what ails them. However, just because a person wants deep pressure doesn't mean that it is appropriate. Use the reflection question below to rehearse possible responses that could be given in this circumstance. Preparing possible answers ahead of time will increase the chances of you giving an intelligent reply.

Reflection Space

A client with stage 4 prostate cancer with mets in the ribs and left ilium has a sore back and strongly requests that you "get in there" with deep pressure. Prior to cancer, this man was a firefighter. His muscle tone is still good. List three possible replies that you could give him regarding the desire for deep pressure.

Final Thoughts:

When I started at OHSU there wasn't a manual to instruct me on how to massage people with cancer. Nurses were the main source of information. Many times I would ask a question, only to be told to "Use your common sense." What they didn't realize is that common sense is based on a deep well of clinical knowledge, a knowledge I didn't have at the time. Clinical decision-making and common sense is dependent on understanding the pathological process of the diseases as well as on how the treatments affect the patient. Good intention and intuition are not enough, not by half. Don't be fooled into thinking they are. The Holy Grail of clinical decision-making involves a combination of three things:

- The therapist's clinical knowledge.
- Verbal information from the client.
- The ability of the therapist to notice subtle signals from the client. This is often identified as intuition, but really it is something much more tangible and conscious. It is a form of non-verbal communication.

Chapter 8

The New Normal:
The Role of Massage During Recovery

For a long time there was not enough discernment between the needs of the patient in treatment and those of the client in recovery. We as educators and therapists often applied the same standards to both groups of people. However, with time, we've seen that as people recover from cancer treatment, we as practitioners need to adjust along with them.

This chapter of MH3 is focused on the recovery period, which includes long-term side effects. These are the side effects that start during treatment and continue on afterwards. Most especially, there is an emphasis in this chapter on exercises that address the risk for lymphedema. Lymphedema can begin during the recovery period or at any time thereafter.

Following are new terms needed for this chapter.

Exercise 1: **Flash cards**

Make flash cards of the following words with the definition or description on the back.

- Axillary web syndrome
- Collagen
- Cording
- DIEP flap
- Fibrin
- Fibrosis
- Free flap

- Late effects
- Long-term side effects
- LT flap
- Lymphedema
- Necrosis
- Neovascularization
- Pain syndrome

- Pedicle flap
- Positive margins
- Post-mastectomy pain syndrome
- Radiation fibrosis
- TRAM flap

Before we begin on other exercises, test yourself on the material in MH3.

Test Yourself

Fill-in: Use the following words to complete the sentences below. Each word should be used only once.

- collagen
- lower
- red
- fatigue
- pain
- radiation fibrosis
- groin
- long-term side effects
- late effects
- inflammatory

1. Which side effect do patients report most affects their quality of life even after treatment has ended?
_____.

2. Patients with one lymph node removed from or radiation to the neck, axilla, or _____ are at risk for lymphedema in the affected quadrant.

3. One of the prime guidelines when massaging someone at risk for lymphedema is: do not use massage strokes that cause the skin to become _____ in the quadrant at risk for lymphedema.

4. Someone who has had nodes removed bilaterally from the groin should have gentler massage in the _____ extremities.

5. The adhesions and scarring created from radiation treatment are referred to as
_____.

6. A _____ syndrome is formed when tissue pain and nerve pain converge over time.

7. Scarring is the laying down of fibrin and _____ in response to tissue trauma.

8. _____ are defined in oncology literature as those that begin during treatment and then linger.

9. _____ begin months or years after treatment ends.

10. Deep massage is contraindicated in a quadrant at risk for lymphedema because it can trigger the _____ process.

True-False: Place a T next to those statements that are true and an F next to those that are false. Rewrite the false statements so that they are true.

1. Over time, radiated tissue can be affected by necrosis, fibrosis, and edema, all side effects of vascular injury.

2. As soon as the redness of radiation treatment has faded from the skin, it is helpful to do deep massage in the area to flush toxins that have built up from radiation.

3. Lymphedema risk stops five years after treatment ends.

4. Massage practitioners may be part of a client's detoxification program, however, the process should be overseen by a health care provider with experience and training.

5. Radiated tissues can become shortened and brittle. Deep tissue massage will help lengthen them.

6. If a client is going to detoxify, it is best done immediately after treatment ends to hasten the healing process.

7. Breast reconstruction is a complex procedure. Approval should be obtained from the plastic surgeon before resuming massage in the surgical areas.

8. Cording is the result of frequent IV catheterizations.

9. Cording is best resolved by heat, stretching and deep massage.

10. Deeper types of scar work, such as stripping or cross fiber friction, are contraindicated if the area has been radiated.

Inching Forward

Many clients and therapists belong to the school of "No Pain, No Gain," which has many campuses around the world. A variation of this method is the university of "If a Little Bit is Good, More Must be Even Better." I myself am a graduate of the institute of "Less is More." One aspect of this approach is to *inch forward* rather than to leap back if the pressure is too great. It is a more common sense approach with all clients, but especially with people who are recovering from medical treatment.

The pressure level for many people can increase as they regain their vigor. However, in the early days of recovery, massage sessions for most people will still include the lighter pressures of levels 1 and 2 with some moderate level 3 pressure being added in as clients are able to tolerate it. The balance between *being* and *doing* starts to shift a little bit. And yet, therapists still need to be mindful of not trying to do too much, too soon.

0/1	Off the body or Light touch	• Energy technique or light touch • Skin contact • Nurturing • Slow • Full hand • As if contacting a ripe PEACH	Severe side effects:	– Blood clot – Bone mets or osteoporosis – Bruising – Edema – End of life – Fatigue – Fever – Fragile – Nausea – Neuropathy – Trauma
2	Superficial muscle	• Contact with superficial muscle • Nurturing • Slow • Full hand • As if gently and slowly washing a PLUM	Moderate side effects:	– Bone mets or osteoporosis – Bruising risk – Fatigue – In-treatment – LE risk – Neuropathy – Trauma
3	Slightly firm	• Slightly firm muscle contact • Inch forward • Not forceful • Not ambitious • As if massaging a TANGERINE	Improving side effects:	– Increased energy – Ready to find "new normal" – Significantly recovered from Tx

Try This: **Doing and being**

Doing and being each has a different feeling. See what you notice about the way in which the two intentions affect your touch.

Intention affects touch—doing v. being

Without telling your partner of your intention, first massage a part of their body with the goal to *fix* it. Do this for a couple of minutes and then slowly come to a stop and remove your hands from their body. After a breath or two, return your hands to the same area, but this time your intent is to just *be with* that part of the body as you give bodywork. Without telling your partner what the two intentions were, ask them to report any differences they noticed.

More is sometimes just more, not better.

—Amy Thurmond, M.D.

Reflection Space

When you tried to *fix* your partner, what did you notice about your own body, hand position, posture, emotions, and thoughts? Were there any differences when you allowed that area of the body to just *be* as it was, not wishing it to be any different? Did you partner report any differences between the intentions?

Inching forward is a concept that can be applied to clients we see over time, such as the one who has a session every two weeks or even every four. The therapist who works in a spa often only sees a client once. There is no inching them forward over time.

Test Yourself

Some conditions lend themselves to inching forward, others don't. Underline the conditions below, which *often* improve over time and might allow for an increased level of demand once treatment is finished. (There are two conditions that I would not underline.)

- lymphedema risk
- fatigue
- incision site
- pain
- radiation fibrosis
- osteoporosis
- cording
- CIPN

Lymphedema Review

Lymphedema risk was one of the above conditions that is not suitable for increasing the level of demand over time. This topic could have been addressed in Chapter 9, however, it was placed in this chapter so as to bring it to the reader's attention sooner rather than later. Lymphedema can occur at any time following lymph node removal or radiotherapy, most especially when the clusters of nodes in the neck, axilla or groin are involved.

Below are a variety of review questions and exercises to deepen your knowledge of this very important topic.

Exercise 2: Adjustments for lymphedema risk

Which of the following actions should be avoided by people at risk for lymphedema? (Underline the correct answers. There are three of them.)

Heat to the affected quadrant.

Exercise.

Blood pressure and injections to the affected side.

Light to moderate pressure massage to the affected side.

Muscle strain.

Cuts, abrasions, paper cuts, insect bites, airline trips.

Exercise 3: **Make a list**

Lymphedema side effects:

List four possible side effects of lymphedema. (Look at the top of page 206 in MH3.)

1.	
2.	
3.	
4.	

When massaging someone at risk for lymphedema:

List the four adjustments (presented on page 208 in MH3) that should be made to the affected quadrant.

1.	
2.	
3.	
4.	

What is the relationship between vigorous massage and lymphedema?

(Three reasons are listed near the bottom of page 207 in MH3.)

1.	
2.	
3.	

Diagramming Lymphedema Risk

Mr. D was treated for melanoma. The only treatment he received was surgical excision of the cancer in the left lower leg, which included a sentinel node biopsy (four nodes) in the groin. He has lymphedema in the lower leg that waxes and wanes. Below, Image A shows the quadrant at risk for lymphedema from the front. Image B indicates, through the use of arrows, which direction massage strokes should be given.

Quadrant at risk for lymphedema—Client D.

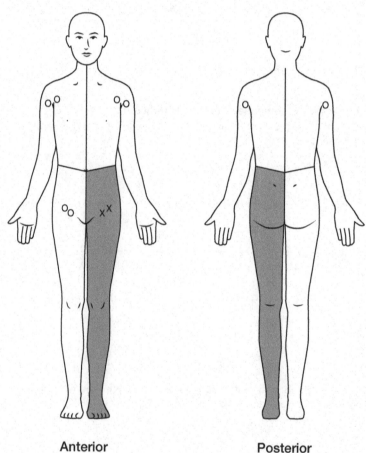

Anterior   Posterior

X = affected nodes
O = unaffected, working nodes

Direction of strokes when massaging Client D's legs.

Image B

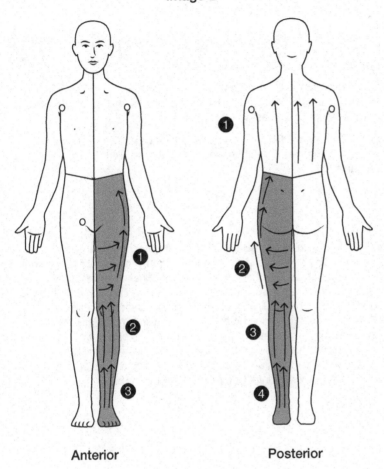

Anterior   Posterior

X = affected nodes
O = unaffected, working nodes

The following guidelines are observed:

1. Start at the proximal segment of the limb, section 1.

2. Stroke toward the working nodes.

3. Stroke only toward the heart.

Pause...and prepare

Make two photocopies of this sample form:

- **Appendix 6, Body Map Worksheet**

Exercise 4: **Diagramming lymphedema risk—Client E**

Let's diagram the lymphedema risk for Client E.

Copy #1: Using the Body Map Worksheet, place Xs and Os to indicate the affected (X) and non-affected (O) clusters of nodes, and shade the quadrant at risk for lymphedema as was done in Image A.

Copy #2: Using the Body Map Worksheet, place arrows to diagram the massage stroke directions that should be used for Client E in the upper quadrants.

Client E

Medical History:

Client E is a 50-year-old female diagnosed with high-grade DCIS ER+/PR+ of the left breast. Her primary care physician referred her to a surgeon who performed a lumpectomy three months ago, which left positive margins. Ten lymph nodes were biopsied during the procedure. She was advised by the surgeon to undergo a double mastectomy, however, she chose to seek a second opinion and decided on a re-excision by a different surgical team. This resulted in clean margins. Immediately following surgery, she was given 33 radiation treatments to her left breast over 45 days. A month after finishing radiation, she began an estrogen suppressing medication, Femara. Client E was previously under the care of a physical therapist for post-surgical and post-radiation side effects—decrease in range of motion, loss of function, and pain due to mild arthritis and bursitis, both of which she believes existed before her cancer diagnosis but were made more painful as a result of the treatments.

Medications *(past and current)*:

(past)

- Femara
- Flexeril
- trazadone

(current)

- Zetia
- acetaminophen

Side effects of treatment and disease:

- **Muscle hypertonicity and fascial binding in left anterior and lateral shoulder**—due to surgery and external beam radiotherapy.
- **Joint pain and bursitis in left shoulder**—worsened due to positioning during surgery and radiation treatment.
- **Pain, moderate but constant (rated 5 out of 10) in left lateral upper arm**—possibly referral pain from tissue binding in left chest.
- **Fatigue**—could be due to hormonal changes and radiation side effects.
- **Insomnia**—possibly due to hormone imbalance.

Pause...and prepare

Make a photocopy of each:

- Appendix 3, Massage Session Planning Worksheet
- Appendix 4, Medications Worksheet

Exercise 5: *Planning the massage session — Client E*

Let's plan the entire massage session for Client E.

Review the medical history and side effects of Client E. As you read and study the information:

1. Summarize her cancer treatment history at the top of the **Massage Session Planning Worksheet**.

2. List her *possible* pressure, site and positioning needs.

3. List Client E's drugs and chemotherapies on the **Medications Worksheet**. Using reliable resources, list the reason for taking each drug, and its common side effects.

4. Is there any information from the **Medications Worksheet** that might be relevant to planning the massage session? If so, list it on the **Massage Session Planning Worksheet**.

Ethics Dilemma

A client with lymphedema due to the side effects of breast cancer surgery is being seen by a physical therapist (PT) for the condition. The client has now been discharged from physical therapy and the PT has referred the client to you for continued lymphedema management. You've only had a two-day weekend course in working with the undamaged lymphatic system. Should you take this client on? Why or why not?

Reflection Space

Reflect on the choice you would make and why.

Final Thoughts

A favorite book of mine is *God's Hotel* by Victoria Sweet. Central to Dr. Sweet's story of Laguna Honda Hospital is the wisdom of the 13th century physician, musician, and nun, Hildegard of Bingen. Hildegard took a gardener's approach to the body, not a mechanic's or a computer programmer's. She did not focus down to the cellular level of the body; instead, she stood back from her patient and looked around. "She manipulated and rebalanced the inner and outer environment of her patient. She did so slowly, like a gardener, by fussing and fiddling, doing a little of this and a little of that. Then she waited to see what would happen. Which is to say that she followed the patient's body; she did not lead."

In contemporary parlance Hildegard's approach would be referred to as client-centered. Too often, however, we modern practitioners shift into being therapist-centered. We become tempted by the multitude of techniques available to us, especially when working with a person who has completed his cancer treatment. Slow is not an easy concept for the present day practitioner. The infinite patience and sensitivity needed goes against the very core of contemporary existence. However, it is worth remembering who won the race between the tortoise and the hare.

Chapter 9

Living Beyond Cancer:
Considerations for Survivors

Officially, the term *survivor* applies to all people with cancer or a history of it. However, for the purposes of this chapter, survivorship is set apart from the treatment, recovery, and end-of-life periods. More closely defining the period in this way is helpful for us as massage therapists in learning how to make adjustments that might be necessary for clients in the post-recovery phase.

In many ways, it is easier to massage people who are in treatment or even in the immediate recovery period. The range of massage possibilities for those who are living beyond the recovery period is much broader and, therefore, more complex for us as practitioners. Some clients achieve a nearly complete recovery and need minimal adjustments to their sessions. Others need continued adjustments for the remainder of their lives. And some develop late effects over time. Late effects are those conditions that appear months or even years following treatment. A client may travel for years on an apparent upward trajectory toward improvement but eventually be affected by late effects. It is the goal of this chapter to make therapists aware of the possibilities that may happen down the road.

This chapter of MH3 is very dense with information. A number of tests and exercises are presented to help you solidify the knowledge and vocabulary components of working with clients at this stage.

Exercise 1: Flash cards

Make flash cards of the following words with the definition or description on the back.

- No evidence of disease (NED)
- Primary cancer
- Progression
- Recurrence
- Relapse
- Remission
- Second cancer
- Survivor

Test Yourself: Surgery

True-False: Place a T next to all true statements and an F next to those that are false. Correct all false statements and re-write them so that they are true. Most false statements can be corrected in more than one way.

1. Late effects appear after treatment ends rather than during treatment.

2. Recurrence refers to the redevelopment of a primary cancer.

3. Cancer that continues to spread is referred to as a relapse.

4. A second cancer is one in which the cancer has spread to distant sites in the body.

5. Radiotherapy can kill cancer cells, but it can also contribute to the development of second cancers.

6. Cancer survivors have a lower rate of osteoporosis than the general population of the same age.

7. People who have had breast, prostate or ovarian cancer run the highest risk of developing osteoporosis.

8. The main symptom of low bone density is achiness in the bones.

9. Certain chemotherapies can contribute to the development of second cancers.

10. A person who receives radiation therapy for head and neck cancer might develop an adrenal dysfunction later in life.

11. Fatigue can be a lifelong problem for many who receive cancer treatments.

12. Radiotherapy for prostate cancer may lead to problems of the urinary tract or sexual dysfunction.

13. Radiation treatment for breast cancer can, in later years, cause the person to be short of breath.

14. Leukemias are always a primary cancer.

15. Some cancer cells develop a resistance to treatment.

Becoming Aware: **The effect of words**

One of the considerations for a person living beyond cancer is the fact that the disease may return. The awareness of this chance may lie below the surface of consciousness but bleeds through in quiet ways. The same may be true for you as a therapist. How do the terms used to describe these possibilities affect you?

Sit in a restful place, close your eyes, take a few breaths, rest for a few moments and then have someone read the following words or read them to yourself, one at a time, with ample space in between each word (at least two minutes). Notice the responses that occur in your body. Is your breathing, the temperature of your body, or your sense of openness affected? Do you pull away or lean into the word? There is no correct response, only awareness.

- Recurrence
- No evidence of disease
- Survivor
- Remission

A full contact massage is one in which the therapist doesn't pull away from anything, not swelling, not risk of recurrence, not fragile bones, not the possibility of death, nothing. The palms of their hands are fully in contact with the client's body, the soles of their feet are fully connected to the floor, their body leans in toward the client, and their heart embraces it all. This is a full contact massage. It has nothing to do with the amount of pressure used.

—Gayle MacDonald, MS, LMT

Reflection Space

What did you notice about your reactions to each of the above words?

Recurrence

No evidence of disease

Survivor

Remission

Three People Living Beyond Cancer

Cancer treatment often changes a person's pressure preferences. For instance, Sheena and Joan were eight and five years out, respectively, from their treatment for breast cancer. Both are massage therapists and received massage before their cancer diagnosis. Prior to cancer treatment, both preferred a pressure level of 4. Now, both women prefer a level 2 pressure in the upper body and a level 3 pressure in the lower body. A level 4 pressure no longer feels comfortable.

Below are summaries for three different people living beyond cancer, each of whom has no evidence of disease. After you read each synopsis, answer the questions below.

Exercise 1: **Short answer**

Ralph

Ralph is eight years post-treatment from colorectal cancer. At the time, he had six cycles of chemotherapy and six weeks of external beam radiation. He is an active 76-year-old, takes no medication, and experiences no physical conditions except swelling in the calves and ankles.

1. What overall pressure would you use for this client, and why?

2. Are there areas of the body where you would use less pressure?

3. Describe in detail how you would massage Ralph's legs. Where would you begin the strokes? In what direction would the strokes go?

Sarah

Sarah started treatment for acute myeloid leukemia four years ago, which included six cycles of chemotherapy over a three-month period. This did not control the disease, so she was given high-dose chemotherapy and a stem cell transplant. At present Sarah is affected by GVHD to the skin, which is treated with 10 mg of prednisone. The skin presents as rashy, itchy, blotchy, with patchy red spots on the chest. Her ferritin level is high, for which she has maintenance phlebotomy every month. The client's energy is approximately 40% of pre-treatment levels on average. She has mild numbness in her fingers and a tendency to swell in the ankles and right knee.

1. What overall pressure would you use, and why?

2. Are there areas where you would use less pressure?

3. Are there areas you might avoid?

Maria

Eight years ago Maria was diagnosed with stage 2 breast cancer of the right breast. Treatment consisted of a mastectomy, including the removal of 13 axillary lymph nodes, eight cycles of chemotherapy, and 30 external beam radiation treatments. All of this took place over a nine-month time span. Maria chose to have breast reconstruction using the TRAM flap procedure. As part of that, a mesh netting was placed in the abdomen. At this point in time, Maria describes her energy as 100%. She has CIPN in her left toes, requiring gentle pressure. The range of motion in her left shoulder and chest is reduced because of surgery and radiotherapy. She is very vigilant about the health of the treated quadrant in terms of lymphedema precautions. Occasionally when she is over active, the arm and the area around the backside of the bra will feel full. This is managed with self-MLD, elevation of the arm and rest. Other remaining side effects are shortness of breath due to fibrosis in the right lung. As well, the site in which the PORT-A-CATH® (port) was placed for chemotherapy is emotionally sensitive. Occasionally Maria will be reminded of the experiences surrounding the port and become tearful. Because of the TRAM flap procedure, Maria has reduced core strength, which means that moving from supine to vertical or supine to prone requires a few extra maneuvers.

1. Based on the information above, what overall, general pressure would you use with Maria? Why? *(Notice "Maria's Body Map" in the section following this. It will give you clues as to overall general pressure.)*

2. Are there areas of the body where you would reduce the pressure?

3. How would you massage her treated quadrant? Describe it in detail. Where would you begin the strokes? In what direction would you stroke? What pressure would you use?

Maria's Body Map—Planning Pressure Use

Below is a body map for Maria using the numbers and gray shading that coincide with the Pressure Guidelines: 1=peach, 2=plum, and 3=tangerine. She, too, likes different pressures to different parts of her body. A 2 pressure is used in the upper left quadrant because of lymphedema risk, in the belly because of the mesh netting, and the head because of personal preference. A 1 pressure is preferred on her left toes due to CIPN. The numbers and shades help us to get a visual of that.

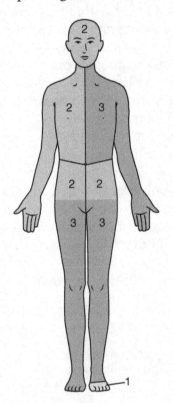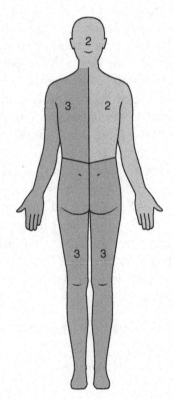

Pause...and prepare

Make a photocopy of:
- **Appendix 6, Body Map Worksheet**

Exercise 2: Client A's Body

Return to Client A in Appendix 5a. Use her medical history to create a body map that shows the various pressures she might need. If possible, use colored pencils that coincide with the Pressure Guidelines.

Discerning the Difference Between Symptoms

In the earlier section, Three People Living Beyond Cancer, examples were presented of people who were living full lives despite experiencing long-term side effects and late effects. At some point in the future, they might develop other late effects, have a recurrence, develop a second cancer, or mature into a ripe old age with the same complaints of anyone who is elderly.

People's responses to the possibilities held by the future are diverse. Some push the potentials as far into the background as possible, others are very vigilant about their health, and some are cavalier. Discerning the difference between symptoms that could be related to cancer or its treatments and those caused by other conditions is not the responsibility of the massage practitioner. Our job is to be aware of the symptoms of late effects, recurrence, or a new second cancer, and suggest that client contacts their health care provider when such symptoms are present.

One practitioner failed to recognize that a client's neck pain might not be muscular in nature but could instead be caused by cancer spreading to the bones. He gave her 11 treatments trying to eliminate the neck pain. The pain only became worse, at which time the client said she was going to stop the bodywork treatments and see her primary care doctor. Scans soon showed that the pain was the result of breast cancer that had metastasized to her cervical spine.

Let's do some short answer exercises to deepen our retention of this information.

Exercise 3: Make a list

Adult survivors of childhood cancers develop many late effects as they mature. List five common side effects that may develop as adults.

1.	
2.	
3.	
4.	
5.	

List five contributing factors to the development of osteoporosis for those treated for cancer.

1.	
2.	
3.	
4.	
5.	

List three possible causes of radiation-induced peripheral neuropathy.

1.	
2.	
3.	

What are some non-specific symptoms of cancer that should be on our radar? List five from the Information Box on page 244 in MH3.

1.	
2.	
3.	
4.	
5.	

Ethics dilemma

A worried massage therapist emailed me with this dilemma, which had become very personal for her on that particular day.

"I've been practicing massage for four years but have not been trained in oncology massage. After an incident that occurred today, I will be seeking out training. A client who has been in remission for almost two years from non-Hodgkins lymphoma was booked in with me. Five years ago she had breast cancer, including the removal of two lymph nodes and radiation therapy. I gently advised the client that I would need a doctor's note to give her massage. When I was in school, we were taught to do that for all active cancer patients, as well as anyone who has had lymph nodes removed, a doctor's clearance was required. The client today became very upset. She said that she had received massage before and was fine. In fact, it was even at the same place where I work. She cried and walked out. I felt so horrible, but I tend to err on the side of caution in these cases because I don't want to hurt anyone.

I would appreciate any advice you can give me going forward on how to handle this kind of a situation. How can I tell a cancer survivor that I can't massage them without making them feel horrible about it? Would practitioners who haven't received additional training in oncology massage be ethically correct in massaging a cancer survivor or someone living with cancer?"

Reflection Space

How would you answer this therapist's questions?

Final Thoughts

Long-term survival of cancer is becoming a reality. With this good news also comes the challenge to understand the implications for the physical, emotional, social and economic needs of patients and their families. It requires us, as part of their wellness team, to be realistic about lingering side effects or the possibility of re-diagnosis, and yet not be held hostage by the dire possibilities. At each stage of the cancer experience, we are tasked with learning to be present with life exactly as it is, not wishing things were any different.

Chapter 10

Side Effects of Cancer:
Disease-Related Adjustments

Planning a massage session, at first, is done in layers. Gathering the information is a bit like an archeological dig. A person with active cancer will have a list of the side effects from treatment, post treatment, and for many, there will be the by-products of the disease itself. These later effects are the focus of this chapter.

Exercise 1: Flash cards

Make flash cards of the following words with the definition or description on the back.

- Anorexia

- Ascites

- Bone metastases

- Cachexia

- Compression neuropathy

- Dyspnea

- Electrolytes

- Hypercalcemia

- Hyperkalemia

- Hyperphosphatemia

- Hypocalcemia

- Osteolysis

- Spinal cord compression syndrome

- Tumor lysis syndrome

Test Yourself

Fill-in: Use the following words to complete the sentences below. Each word should be used only once. (There are a few red herrings thrown in.)

- liver
- hypercalcemia
- neutropenic
- lung
- blood clots
- dyspnea
- hyperkalemia
- ovarian
- tumor lysis syndrome
- anorexia
- ascites
- osteolysis
- prostate

1. _____ occurs because of the break-down of cancer cells, which releases the contents of the cells.

2. One of the main causes of _____ is an increase in the amount of calcium released from bones as they undergo lysis due to bone cancers or bone metastases.

3. A _____ fever is related to a low white blood count.

4. The majority of bone metastases occur most often with advanced cases of breast and _____ cancers.

5. The medical term for breathing difficulty is _____.

6. Too much potassium in the blood stream is known as _____.

7. Nausea and vomiting is typically associated with cancer treatment, but it can also be a result of electrolyte imbalance, constipation, or _____ tumors.

8. After infection, _____ are the leading cause of death in cancer patients.

9. _____ is a condition that often accompanies advanced cancers of the abdomen, such as liver, ovarian, colon and pancreatic.

10. The break down or disappearance of bone tissue is referred to as _____.

Exercise 1: **Creating a sentence**

Use the following terms in a sentence that demonstrates an understanding of some clinical aspect of the condition as it relates to people with cancer.

Example: **Ascites**   *The patient was having breathing difficulties as a result of ascites.*

Bone metastases	
Electrolyte imbalance	
Nerve impingement	
Osteolysis	
Spinal cord compression syndrome	
Cachexia	
Hematological	
Hypocalcemia	
Carcinogen	

Exercise 2: **Side effects—treatment, disease, or both?**

Many side effects are mainly the result of treatment and others are caused most often by the disease. Place an X in each box that is true.

Side effect	Treatment-related	Disease-related
Example: Alopecia	X	
1. Anemia		
2. Ascites		
3. Bone mets		
4. Breathing difficulty		
5. Constipation		
6. Edema		
7. Fever		
8. Fibrosis		
9. Hand-foot syndrome		
10. Headache		
11. Hypercalcemia		
12. Lymphedema		

13. Nausea		
14. Neutropenia		
15. Nerve impingement		
16. Peripheral neuropathy		
17. Osteoporosis		
18. Thrombocytopenia		
19. Vital organ complications		
20. VTE (DVT)		

Exercise 3: Make a list

List five symptoms that can occur when calcium is out of balance.

1.	
2.	
3.	
4.	
5.	

List five causes of headache in people with cancer.

1.	
2.	
3.	
4.	
5.	

List five advanced cancers that increase the risk of developing a blood clot.

1.	
2.	
3.	
4.	
5.	

Exercise 4: Side effects and specific cancers

Specific cancers are associated with certain side effects. This has only to do with the disease process, rather than being caused by treatment. For instance, people with liver cancer can be affected by easy bruising, however, the disease of breast cancer does not cause this same effect. Nausea also can be connected to liver cancer, but it is generally not a by-product of leukemia.

In this exercise, place an X in the box if the side effect has a relationship to any of the six specific cancers listed at the top.

Side effect	leukemia	breast	ovarian	prostate	lung	colon
Example: 1. Anemia	X					
2. Bone fragility						
3. Bowel changes, e.g., constipation, diarrhea						
4. Fatigue						
5. Fever						
6. Nausea						
7. Neutropenia						
8. Thrombocytopenia						
9. VTE (DVT)						

Pause...and prepare

Make a copy of the following forms from the Appendices:

- **Appendix 3, Massage Session Planning Worksheet**
- **Appendix 4, Medications Worksheet**

Exercise 5: *Planning a massage session–Client F*

Review the medical history and side effects of Client F. As you read and study the information, list her possible pressure, site and positioning needs on the Massage Session Planning Worksheet. Use the Medications Worksheet to record the common side effects from Client E's medications.

Client F

Medical History

Client F is a 68-year-old woman with stage 3 multiple myeloma. She was diagnosed 15 years ago. The original treatment was chemotherapy for a year followed the next year by a stem cell transplant and four more years of chemotherapy. Client F was able to be off chemotherapy for four years but following a relapse has been on Revlimid for maintenance for the past six years. She's received radiation to the thoracic spine in an attempt to control the myeloma in that area. Over time she has fractured her fibula, ribs and various vertebrae due to weakened bone, a result of the disease. Four years ago she had a kyphoplasty due to collapsed vertebrae. Client F is immunosuppressed and is on medication for prevention of shingles and pneumonia.

Despite fatigue, peripheral neuropathy in the lower legs and feet and poor balance, this client is an active woman. She takes classes at the local university, participates in cultural events, attends yoga twice a week and Neuromuscular Integrative Action (NIA) twice a week, and a monthly support group.

Medications *(current)*:
- Aredia
- famotidine
- losartan
- Lexapro
- Lyrica
- Mepron
- Oxycontin
- Revlimid
- Valtrex

Side effects of treatment and disease:
- **Fatigue**—due to the disease and chemotherapy, both of which lower red blood cell count.
- **Immunosuppression**—due to lowered white blood cell count, a side effect of chemo and multiple myeloma.
- **Easy bruising**—due to the disease and chemotherapy, both of which lower her platelets.
- **Peripheral neuropathy**—(CIPN) due to chemotherapy.
- **Bone lesions**—due to multiple myeloma.
- **Bone instability**—due to multiple myeloma.
- **Nerve pain**—due to CIPN.
- **Pain**—related to CIPN.
- **Depression**—due to circumstances.
- **Acid reflex**—due to aging.

Ethics Dilemma

A client omits his cancer history to you because he is afraid you will turn him away. Several massages later you find out he is under a doctor's care for a recurrent cancer.

Reflection Space

What would your reaction be? How would you approach this situation with the client? Perhaps you've experienced this already. If so, were you happy with your response? Would you change it in any way?

Final Thoughts

Too often, cancer seems to appear in capital letters—CANCER—followed by an exclamation point—! The word *cancer* stops people in their tracks when they see or hear it. They hold their breath and freeze for a moment. Yes, cancer is intense, but so is diabetes, kidney disease, MRSA, and macular degeneration. Cancer does not have to engender fear in massage therapists, nor define clients.

It is a common adage that "if you have your health, you have everything." The opposite side of that belief is that without your health, you have nothing. A person's health status doesn't define them. We are all more than our health. After working with the exercises in this chapter, it is easy to get caught up in the clinical milieu, but always, we must come back to the person, not the disease.

Chapter 11

Being is Enough:
Comforting Touch at the End of Life

The landscape at the end of life is very foreign to the modern-day person because dying and death has become a medical event. Several generations ago, death, like birth, happened at home. The care for and stages of dying were more familiar. I'm not advocating a return to the old days, but I am suggesting that it has become unfamiliar ground that we must reacquaint ourselves with.

People who are dying from cancer are as diverse as any other group of people with a cancer history. Their capacities, clinical profiles, and massage requests vary greatly. Some people remain fairly active until the last few weeks. My first hospice patient, for example, drove herself to her massage appointments until two weeks prior to death. Others decline slowly over several years.

The topic of comforting touch at the end of life could fill an entire book. Please seek additional reading and trainings on this subject. The exercises and quizzes in this chapter barely scratch the surface.

Test Yourself

True-False: Place a T next to all true statements and an F next to those that are false. Correct all false statements and re-write them so that they are true. Some false statements can be corrected in more than one way.

1. Hospice is not necessarily a place, but is a philosophy of care.

2. Touch is more welcome at the end of life than at any other time.

3. A person who is dying cannot be damaged any further. Therefore, pressure precautions are no longer an issue.

4. Continue to greet people who are no longer conscious. Explain who you are and what your purpose is in being there.

5. Sitting on the bed is appropriate with hospice clients.

6. The body may stiffen as a sign that the person does not want to be touched.

7. The bowels nearly always become sluggish as a result of narcotic medications. Gentle massage can often be given to help the bowels move.

8. Listening and receiving the person exactly as he is are the best tools the massage therapist has.

9. At the end of life, people have fewer positioning needs.

10. When massaging people nearing the end of life, the consultation process should be carried out with a family member rather than the client.

11. Touch sessions at the end of life should be longer in duration but with gentler pressure.

12. People in the later stages of life tend to prefer massage to isolated parts of the body.

13. The term palliative care can be used interchangeably with hospice care.

14. Patients with a stage 1 pressure sore (reddened but intact skin) will benefit by massage directly to the area.

15. Hearing is the first sense to go as the end of life approaches.

Birth and Death: Comparable Stages

The stages of dying can be understood by comparing them to the stages of pregnancy, labor and birth—quickening, lightening, active labor and the moment of death.

Exercise 1: **Short answer**

Part A: Quickening

Briefly define quickening as it relates to pregnancy and the dying process.

List three signs that a person may be entering this stage.

1.

2.

3.

Part B: Lightening

Briefly define lightening as it is used in obstetrics and end-of-life care.

List five of the signs associated with this phase.

1.
2.
3.
4.
5.

Part C: Active labor

Briefly describe active labor as it relates to birth and death.

List three changes that would indicate the patient has entered this phase.

1.

2.

3.

Part D: Moment of death

Briefly describe how the moment of birth and moment of death can be similar.

List three changes that occur at the moment of death.

1.

2.

3.

Becoming Aware: **Being present with the dying**

The following questions will help you become aware of your own thoughts about working with the dying. As you quietly reflect on them, allow yourself to be free of judgment, accepting what surfaces without analysis or interpretation. Once you have answered, take some time to reflect on your responses. Notice how your experiences with or ideas about dying have shaped you.

Reflection Space

I believe that dying…

When I give a massage to someone who is dying or imagine myself doing it, I feel…

Reflection Space

As I work with a dying person, or imagine it, my body feels...

When I am present with a dying person, or imagine it, and not focused on an outcome or their disease process, I feel or think...

What would be your hopes for yourself in working with someone who is dying?

Exercise 2: **Medications for symptom management**

Once a person stops pursing treatment, medications are given mostly for symptom management. Below are some of the common classifications used in this pursuit.

Type of drug	Reason for use	Examples
Narcotics	Pain, dyspnea, sleep	oxycodone, dilaudid
Anti-anxietal	Anxiety, dyspnea	diazepam, lorazepam
Neuroleptic	Delirium	haloperidol
Anti-emetic	Nausea and vomiting	metoclopramide, cannabis
Anti-cholinergics/anti-histamines	To reduce saliva and lung secretions	atropine, Levsin, scopolamine
Laxatives/suppositories	Constipation	senna, lactulose, magnesium

Pause...and prepare

Make a copy of the following form from the Appendices:
- **Appendix 4, Medications Worksheet**

Exercise 3: **Medications research**

Research the following often-prescribed drugs or treatments and record your findings on the Medications Worksheet:
- oxygen
- acetaminophen (Tylenol)
- oxycodone (Oxycontin)
- lorazepam (Ativan)
- haloperidol (Haldol)
- ondansetron (Zofran)
- atropine (Atropen)
- senna

Make a copy of the following forms from the Appendices:
- **Appendix 3, Massage Session Planning Worksheet**
- **Appendix 4, Medications Worksheet**

Exercise 4: Planning a massage session—Client G

Review the medical history and side effects of Client G. As you read and study the information, list his possible pressure, site and positioning needs on the Massage Session Planning Worksheet. Use the Medications Worksheet to record the common side effects from Client G's medications.

Client G

Medical History:
Client G is an 83-year-old man diagnosed with end-stage colon cancer. This cancer is a late effect from cobalt radiation treatment for testicular cancer in 1949. In his 70's he had 12 strokes, none of which impacted him significantly because he was able to get medical attention immediately. Testicular cancer was the first of five primary cancers in his life. Several decades later he experienced stage 2 bladder cancer, which was treated with external beam radiation. Free of cancer for four years, he was then diagnosed with stage 2 prostate cancer, which was treated with external beam radiation. Cancer-free for approximately three years, his bladder cancer returned and he was treated again with radiation. Approximately two years into his remission from his second round of bladder cancer he was diagnosed with thyroid cancer. This was treated surgically and he was considered cured. Several years later his prostate cancer returned. This time, treatment included radiation and an oral hormonal medication. After several months of treatment, he was considered cancer free and cured for several years until his diagnosis of colon cancer.

Client G is a Marine Corps veteran who was surgically treated many years ago for shrapnel wounds in the abdomen. The scars in this area are not physically uncomfortable as much as spiritually and psychologically painful. As a former Marine, Client G doesn't identify with the word "pain." Instead, the term "discomfort" has to be used.

Medications (current):
- Coumadin
- oxycodone
- Ativan
- atenolol

Side effects of previous treatments and current disease progression:
- **Alternate diarrhea and constipation**—due to disease progression of colon cancer.
- **Increasing fatigue**—but still physically strong and ambulating, he does not require personal assistance for hygiene or grooming needs.
- **Low back and abdominal pain**—due to colon cancer. The pain is increasing in intensity and frequency, requiring more and larger doses of pain medicine. Finds comfort in reclined position or occasionally supine in bed. Abdomen is also sensitive from shrapnel wounds.
- **Sundowning, agitation, anxiety, disorientation and restlessness**—as dusk approaches, requiring additional comfort measures.
- **Sleep is interrupted**—by dreams in which he finds himself traveling to new places. He awakens disoriented, but gets dressed to go out to see friends. Even if it is 3am.
- **Anxiety and hostility**—occurs as sleep is increasingly disrupted. He has angry outbursts on a regular basis.
- **Skin is extremely fragile**—especially on the hands and arms.
- **Arthritis in hands.**

*In many Muslim cultures,
when you want to ask them how
they're doing, you ask: in Arabic,
Kayf haal-ik? or, in Persian,
Haal-e shomaa chetoreh?
How is your haal?*

*What is this haal
that you inquire about?
It is the transient state of
one's heart. In reality, we ask,
"How is your heart doing at this
very moment, at this breath?"
When I ask, "How are you?" that
is really what I want to know.*

—Omid Safi

Try This: **Open-ended greetings**

Many of the questions used in greeting people, such as "How are you?" are closed-ended and trite, especially when a person has a limited amount of time to live. Practice for a day or two with some of the more meaningful conversational openings listed below.

- What has your morning/afternoon/week been like?
- It's great to see you today. How can I best help you?
- What is your hope for today?

Try these out with those in your every day life: children, partners, workmates or friends. In order to become skilled at new language, we must practice in more relaxed circumstances.

Reflection Space

What did you notice when using open-ended greetings?

Exercise 5: **Make a list**

When a person is dying, they may not be able to communicate verbally.
List five nonverbal signs that they may be uncomfortable (from MH3,
pages 279-80).

1.	
2.	
3.	
4.	
5.	

What are five non-verbal signs that the person is comfortable (from MH3,
page 280)?

1.	
2.	
3.	
4.	
5.	

Try This: **Touch for the dying**

Massage at the end of life can distract the dying person from letting go, bringing their attention back to the body. Touch at this time should be freeing and reassuring, supporting the person as they release into the unknown. How can we touch someone, anyone, in a way that does not hold him back but instead allows freedom?

Try this with a partner. Imagine she is at the very end of life, actively laboring through the end-of-life passageway, a birth canal of sorts. What kind of touch would feel freeing and reassuring?

Reflection Space

Describe what it was like to try giving touch that was freeing. How was it different than your usual session? What was your body position like? Your hands? Your intention?

Ethics Dilemma

Your client is no longer eating or drinking on a regular basis, which is disturbing to his family. They feel if they can keep him eating, he will live longer. When you check in with them before entering the client's room, his daughter asks you to urge him to eat and drink more. You are handed a glass of juice to take in with you to see if you might have better luck than they have getting him to drink something.

Reflection Space

There are many aspects to the above situation: scope of practice, responsibility to the client, possible suggestion to the family, and more. Reflect on these aspects and how you would respond to this situation.

Final Thoughts

In our culture, death is difficult to come to grips with. Ours is a society that, by and large, prefers youth to aging, light rather than dark, summer as opposed to winter, continual growth versus disintegration, fullness rather than emptiness, hope instead of despair. We want to live on only one part of the spectrum instead of through the complete cycle of life and death.

We have come to value productivity above all else. We've bought into the belief in consumerism, which relies on productivity. On the surface, it would seem that productivity is related to youth, light, warmth and optimism; productivity wanes in the dark and cold, in rest and idleness, in old age and death. But the two opposites are inextricably linked. Without idleness, there is no creativity or productivity; without death, there is no life; without winter there is no spring or summer. Every gardener knows that seeds require the fallowness of winter to rest and gather power. Then, in spring they have the energy to break the casing that surrounds them, thrusting their way up through the earth's crust. True power is built by living the complete cycle of life.

Death clears the way for new growth, and we can prepare for it every day by welcoming aging, the dark, the cold, winter, dormancy, rest, disintegration and impermanence. Each of these facets of life gives us a chance to practice being with things exactly as they are, not wishing they were any different. It is this deep belief in the circle of life that allows us to be present with ourselves and others at this most profound moment: death.

In the end these things matter most:

How well did you love?

How fully did you live?

How deeply did you let go?

—Jack Kornfield

Chapter 12

Companions on the Journey:
Who Gives? Who Receives?

Victoria Sweet, author of *God's Hotel*, writes about the root of the word *hospital*, which is *hospitality*. Sweet says, "The essence of hospitality—*hospes*—is that guest and host are identical, if not in the moment, then at some moment. Whatever our current role, it is temporary. With time and the seasons, a host goes traveling and becomes a guest; a guest returns home and becomes a host. That is what the word *hospitality* encodes."

Just as guest and host represent two sides of the same coin, so, too, are therapist and client, nurse and patient, giver and receiver. Each is contained within the other and cannot be separated. For instance, without a receiver there is no giver. Without the client there is no therapist. They are two parts of the same spectrum.

This way of thinking is holistic in nature. It acknowledges healing as an interdependent process in which the client is an equal partner who has medicine to offer the practitioner. They are teacher and expert, in a holistic approach, they are someone who is allowed to feel useful, giving and needed. When patients feel that they belong to the process, symptoms often diminish, become more tolerable, or disappear. As for us, we are more whole and mature companions on the journey when we can also be the novice, the receiver, and the one who is served.

Our desire to work with people who have cancer is often more complex than we realize. Being conscious of the various influences helps to create and maintain a healthy patient-practitioner relationship. In order to achieve this, we must delve into our personal motivations for working with people who are medically complex. The exercises in this chapter are designed to assist with that.

The only gift I have to give
is the ability to receive.
If giving is a gift, and it surely is,
then my gift to you is to allow you
to give to me.

—Jarod Kintz

Holism or Hierarchy?

Our culture values some qualities more than others, such as giving, helping, and being strong. Scant attention is paid to the flip side of these attributes. However, it is important to examine the opposite end of the spectrum. If we only concentrate on being the expert, the giver, or the healthy one, the relationship is hierarchical rather than circular. Hierarchical relationships are based on one person being more powerful than the other. This way of relating leads to feelings of separation, lack of creativity, or burn out.

Exercise 1: Giving and receiving

Part 1: Focus on being the giver. Close your eyes and rest for a moment. Imagine you are with someone affected by cancer. It might be a client, family member or friend, or perhaps it is an imaginary person. Envision the surroundings of the room you are in, the quality of the person's energy, how they are dressed and positioned. See yourself with them. You are there to give them gentle massage. Allow yourself to sink into the vision. Once you can imagine connecting with this person, become aware of what you hope to give through your presence and touch.

Reflection Space

List three gifts you hope to give to this imaginary person.

1.

2.

3.

Part 2: Now, switch gears and focus on receiving. Within this same scenario, notice what this situation gives to you. *(It's ok to receive from clients.)* Another way to think about this question is: Who do you get to be in this situation? Or, are there qualities from the person who is ill that you would like to integrate into your life? When we open to the experience of illness, we see the opportunities within it and no longer see the ill person as a victim to be pitied.

Reflection Space

List three of the gifts you receive from the person in this imaginary moment.

1.

2.

3.

What hinders you from being receptive?

(This exercise could be repeated with a variety of word pairs that represent opposite ends of the spectrum, such as strong and weak, expert and novice, and being and doing.)

Idealizing Clients—Life on a Pedestal

Sometimes we are attracted to working with people who are more fragile because it gives us an opportunity to feel heroic. If we aren't careful, that desire for heroism can be projected onto the person with cancer. Rather than engaging holistically, we've created another kind of a hierarchy. In this version, the client with cancer is held in high esteem as noble and brave, a sacred hero, someone to be idealized. Elevation in this way places a distance between practitioner and patient. Being on a pedestal is exhausting and requires people with cancer to hold themselves together in order that those around them—family, friends, health care providers, and work mates—won't suffer.

Try This: Idealization and pity

We've all been through difficult events in our lives. Very few people, including those with cancer, want to be idealized or pitied because of those events. Notice how either of these states of being affect your presence and touch with a practice partner.

Instructions:

1. Decide who will be the first receiver. The receiver can position himself on the table in any way. Giver and receiver should agree ahead of time upon which part of the body the giver will rest her hands.
2. **Giver:** Prior to resting your hands on your partner's body, take a moment to shift into a place of idealizing the receiver. Then allow your hands to settle onto the receiver as you hold onto a sense of that emotion.
3. Hold that position emotionally and physically for about 90 seconds, then gently lift your hands off.
4. Re-center without speaking.
5. When you are ready, shift into a state of feeling pity for your partner. Replace your hands in the same place.
6. After you finish holding that position emotionally and physically for about 90 seconds, lift your hands away. Share with each other what you noticed about either giving or receiving from the places of idealization and pity.
7. Change places and repeat.

(*Alternative:* Imagine you are a hero who thinks that your partner needs to be saved. How does that affect your touch and presence?)

Reflection Space

What did you notice about the effects of pity and idealization as the giver? And as the receiver?

Giver

Receiver

*I slept and I dreamed that
life is all joy.
I woke and I saw that
life is all service.
I served and I saw that
service is joy.*

—Kahlil Gibran

Fix, Help or Serve?

Rachel Naomi Remen, in several of her writings and speeches, addresses the topic of service, which she describes as a relationship between two equals. "Our service," she states, "serves us as well as others. That which uses us strengthens us. Over time, fixing and helping are draining, depleting. Over time, we burn out. Service is renewing. When we serve, our work itself will sustain us."

Becoming Aware: **The effect of words**

Let's examine how fixing, helping and serving feel different physically and emotionally. Sit in a restful place, close your eyes, take a few breaths, and rest for a moment. Have someone read the following words or read them to yourself, one at a time, with ample space (at least two minutes) in between each word. Notice the responses that occur in your body. Is your breathing, the temperature of your body, your sense of openness or being closed, softness or hardness affected? There is no correct response, only awareness.

- Fix
- Help
- Serve

Reflection Space

What did you notice about the effect each word had on you? How did it affect you physically and emotionally? How would each of these approaches affect the quality of your presence or touch when massaging someone affected by cancer?

Fix

Help

Serve

Client-Therapist Boundaries

Warm sentiments naturally develop between clients and massage therapists, which usually has positive ramifications. Feeling cared for is good for patients' healing. Occasionally, however, there are negative outcomes, such as when a boundary is crossed if therapists are unconsciously trying to meet their own needs. Patients are best able to heal when the focus is on them rather than feeling any need to take care of the therapist.

Exercise 2: **Personal boundaries**

Following are a few questions to think about regarding your personal boundaries with clients:

1. Do you ever have an overwhelming need to be needed and thus build relationships with patients based on this need?
2. How do your personal experiences influence your reactions and impact your ability to form healthy relationships with patients and family?
3. Do you over-extend yourself for certain clients at a personal cost to you?

Reflection Space

Use the space below to explore the three questions listed just above.

Need to be needed

Reflection Space

Use the space below to explore the three questions listed just above.

Personal experiences

Over-extending yourself

Care for Our Own Well-Being

Cancer can be a long journey. A patient's companions must maintain their own equanimity in order to endure. Dan Siegel, MD, pioneer in interpersonal neurobiology, advises that "If you care about others, take care of yourself first." And yet, that recommendation runs counter to the cultural belief that it is better to give than to receive. How then do we navigate these conflicting positions? I don't have the answer because I, too, am in a constant search for the balance between myself and others.

Many years ago, I used Stephen Levine's loving kindness meditation when teaching the hospital classes. The exercise starts by asking the listener to "direct care for our own well-being," to relate to the self with kindness, compassion, and mercy. Most of us noticed how much easier it is to extend those qualities to others rather than to ourselves.

The term *self-care* has been so overused as to become trite. It generally connotes those things we do to take care of ourselves in a physical way, such as good nutrition, exercise, time with family, and activities that bring pleasure. All of these are important, however, let's consider a more profound meaning, a feeling that we matter. The ultimate self-care would be attending to ourselves because at the deepest level we feel that we matter.

Try This: **Mercy and kindness**

For a moment, sit with your eyes closed and send yourself mercy and kindness.

Reflection Space

What was it like to be merciful and kind to yourself? Take your time in writing about it. Perhaps other insights will come to you as you write.

Exercise 3: **Short answer**

On page 311 of the Self-care section in MH3 is a bulleted list of questions that flag the potential for inadequate self-care. If you were going to focus on exploring one of them, which would it be?

List three strategies that appeal to you for exploring this issue, such as journaling, peer supervision, or taking a meditation class. Place a star beside the one you are most likely to use. *(I shall leave it up to you whether you take this further.)*

1.

2.

3.

Final Thoughts

Chapter 13, Companions on the Journey, is the shortest chapter in MH3. However, it is of no less importance than the others. To be sure, our work has a clinical and intellectual side, but our heart-felt presence holds equal, if not greater, weight. Every time I've re-written *Medicine Hands*, I've toyed with the idea of putting this chapter at the beginning of the book to signal its importance.

When teaching classes, I always start with a heart-related exercise. Clinical thinking and skills can be mastered over time, but the heart is always evolving and growing, breaking and expanding, reaching toward infinity. If you work with people who are profoundly ill, you will be attending to your heart for the rest of your life.

Being confronted with the circumstances of cancer over and over again, we, as therapists, develop a desire for things to be different than they are. We wish for clients to be given the all-clear, for parents to be allowed to raise their children, for people to regain their old lives once treatment is over, for this dread disease to be conquered. However, the more we can expand our hearts to allow things to be exactly as they are, the more we can be companions on the journey.

Appendices

Appendix 1 *Sample Letter to Health Care Provider*

Grace Johnson   1234 NE Rancho Ave   Tucson, AZ 87654   480.234.5678   jhands@mymail.com

Dear Dr. Calibri,

Your patient, Karen Smith, has expressed an interest in receiving massage therapy during her cancer treatment. I am writing to outline my experience and the common cautions I use when working with people in cancer treatment.

I am a Licensed Massage Therapist and certified Manual Lymph Drainage practitioner who specializes in cancer care massage. Currently I work part-time at University Hospital providing massage to patients in the Outpatient Cancer Center and the Inpatient Hematology/Oncology unit. I also have a private practice dedicated to serving people with medically complex situations.

Below are the common adjustments I make for people receiving cancer treatment:

- I adjust the pressure for each client depending on their specific treatments and the side effects they are experiencing. Some examples are:
  - Low platelet levels or risk of thrombosis secondary to malignancy, inactivity or cancer treatment. I use gentle pressure that only moves skin and other superficial tissues, *not* deep muscle layers.
  - If there is lymphedema present or a risk of it, I use only minimal pressure on the affected quadrant and modify the direction of my massage strokes. I sometimes incorporate Manual Lymph Drainage into the session.

- When areas of the body are affected by surgery, radiation therapy, IV's, drains, skin conditions, pain, edema or bone involvement, I use gentle pressure and/or may avoid massage to that area until it is healed.

- Positioning may also be adjusted due to such situations as surgical incisions, breast implants, or shortness of breath.

Sincerely,
Grace Johnson, LMT

_____ has my permission to receive massage as described above. Additional concerns are listed below.

_____   _____
Health Care Provider Signature   Date

| Appendix 2 *Sample Massage Benefits List* |

Potential Benefits of Massage for People with Cancer

- Moisturizes the skin and prevents problems such as bedsores or tears in the skin.
- Relieves muscle soreness resulting from prolonged bedrest.
- Increases range of motion.
- Increases relaxation.
- Temporarily decreases edema.
- Sedates or stimulates the nervous system, depending on the modality used.
- Encourages deeper respiration.
- Improves bowel activity.
- Increases alertness and mental clarity.
- Improves sleep.
- Provides short-term pain relief.
- Improves short-term fatigue.
- Stimulates faster wound healing.
- Increases elasticity in areas affected by scars or adhesions.
- Increases effectiveness of other treatments, such as pain medication, physical therapy or medical procedures.
- Increases awareness of stress signals.
- Provides short-term decrease of anxiety.
- Distraction.
- Provides relief from isolation and offers meaningful social interaction.
- Creates a doorway to greater intimacy with family and friends.
- Relieves touch deprivation.
- Provides a forum to express feelings.
- Re-establishes a positive body image.
- Gives patients a sense of participation in the healing process.
- Rebuilds hope.

Appendix 3 *Massage Session Planning* Worksheet 1 of 2

As you read the client profile, slot their health considerations into the appropriate category: pressure, site, or position. Some conditions should be categorized in two and sometimes three of the categories. When planning a session, you won't know the absolute adjustments until you meet the client. At this point, they are possible adjustments.

1. Type of cancer and location _____

2. Date of diagnosis _____

3. Presently in treatment?   No   Yes

If yes, what type? _____

If no, when did treatment end? _____

4. TREATMENT REVIEW: Year

Surgery: No   Yes   Describe _____

_____

Radiation: No   Yes   Area _____

_____

Chemo: No   Yes   Rounds _____

_____

5. REVIEW of SIDE EFFECTS and HEALTH CONSIDERATIONS

Pressure Adjustments:

Systemic pressure adjustments:

What overall pressure would you use for this client?_____
List the reasons:

Continued on page 2

Appendix 3 *Massage Session Planning* Worksheet 2 of 2

Local pressure adjustments:

Site Restrictions:

Areas to be mindful of:

Are there areas on which you *might* use less pressure from the overall pressure listed earlier? List those areas below:

Positioning Adjustments:

6. What further clarifications would you want from this client?

Appendix 4 *Medications* Worksheet

List all of the client's supplements, present medications and chemotherapies, as well as past chemotherapies. Using a drug reference guide or the internet, research the drug, the most likely reason it is prescribed, and the common side effects.

Drug	Reason for prescribing	Common side effects

If you need more space, make sufficient photocopies of this worksheet to accommodate the complete list.

Appendix 5a *Client A: Medical History* Worksheet

Client A

Medical History

Client A is a 48-year-old woman who had been in good health prior to diagnosis. She has slightly elevated blood pressure that is controlled with medication. Eight months ago she discovered a lump in her left breast, which was diagnosed as stage 3, estrogen and progesterone receptor positive (ER+/PR+). She had a mastectomy with 12 lymph nodes removed, followed by six rounds of a chemotherapy regimen referred to as TAC (Taxotere, Adriamycin, and cyclophosphamide) over 18 weeks. During that time, she experienced low white count and low platelets, hair loss, mucositis, loss of appetite, nausea and vomiting the first few days, joint pain and slight neuropathy in a few toes. At this time she received 28 of 33 radiation therapy (RT) treatments to the left chest wall.

Since the surgery, she has had some numbness and prickling sensations under her left arm and in the axilla. Her hair is growing back. Her blood counts are within the normal range. Following surgery her ROM returned fairly quickly, however, the radiation treatment has caused the muscles in the left chest to be tight. Her ROM now is less than it was following surgery. Her left neck and shoulder are also stiff from protecting the area. So far, A, an avid yoga practitioner, shows no signs of lymphedema in the left arm. She continues to be fatigued, although her energy has improved enough to enable her to work from home. At this time she is in survival mode, using her limited energy to work and to provide for her daily needs. She is not in an intimate relationship at this time, which is very upsetting to her. For this reason she enjoys receiving touch through massage.

Medications *(past and current)*:
(past)
- Taxotere
- Adriamycin
- cyclophosphamide
- oxycodone

(current)
- Ambien
- lisinopril
- Zoloft
- tamoxifen

Side effects of treatment and disease:
- **Fatigue**—due to surgery, chemo and radiation and the emotional roller coaster.
- **Extreme tenderness and inflammation**—in treated area.
- **Risk for lymphedema L upper quadrant**—dissection of and RT to nodes in axilla.
- **Reduced ROM in left shoulder**—result of surgery and fibrosis from RT.
- **Numbness and prickling under left arm and axilla**—nerves cut during nodal dissection.
- **Tightness in L chest muscles**—result of surgery but mostly fibrosis and inflammation from RT.
- **Chemo brain**—chemo.
- **Joint pain**—residue from chemotherapy.
- **Peripheral neuropathy in toes**—due to chemotherapy.

Appendix 5b *Client A: Medications* Worksheet

List all of the client's medications and chemotherapies being taken now and during treatment, as well as present supplements. Using a drug reference guide or the internet, research the drug, the most likely reason it is prescribed, and the common side effects.

Drug	Reason for prescribing	Common side effects
(past) Taxotere	Anti-neoplastic derived from the periwinkle plant. Inhibits cell division and reproduction.	Neutropenia, anemia, thrombocytopenia, fluid retention, CIPN, nausea and vomiting, diarrhea, mucositis, alopecia, fatigue, weakness, nail changes, muscle/joint/bone pain, abnormal liver function.
(past) Adriamycin	Anti-neoplastic antibiotic derived from soil fungus. Affects cells at multiple phases of cell cycle.	Neutropenia, anemia, thrombocytopenia, mucositis, alopecia, watery eyes, dark urine, radiation recall, infertility.
(past) cyclophosphamide	Anti-neoplastic derived from mustard gas. Affects cells in the resting phase.	Neutropenia, anemia, thrombocytopenia, mucositis, alopecia, nausea and vomiting, poor appetite, infertility, discoloration of nails or skin, bladder irritation and bleeding. Delayed possibility of developing a hematological cancer.
(past) oxycodone	Pain—narcotic based.	Nausea, vomiting, loss of appetite, dry mouth, light-headedness, dizziness, stomach pain, heartburn, drowsiness, weakness, mood changes, constipation, anxiety, indigestion, trouble sleeping.
(present) lisinopril	Blood pressure.	Cough, dizziness, headache, fatigue, nausea, diarrhea, weakness.
(present) Zoloft	Depression.	Decreased libido, drowsiness, nervousness, insomnia, dizziness, nausea, rash, headache, dizziness, constipation, stomach upset, appetite changes, dry mouth.
(present) tamoxifen	Suppression of hormones that feed breast cancer.	Bone loss, hot flashes, nausea, fatigue, mood swings, depression, headache, thinning hair, constipation, dry skin, loss of libido, fluid retention, vaginal bleeding or discharge; (Rare): blood clot risk, stroke, cataracts, uterine cancer.
(present) Ambien	Sleep	Drowsiness, dizziness, light-headedness, fatigue, loss of coordination, stuffy nose, dry mouth, nose or throat irritation, nausea, constipation, diarrhea, stomach upset, headache

Appendix 5c *Client A: Massage Session Planning* Worksheet 1 of 2

As you read the client profile, slot their health considerations into the appropriate category: pressure, site, or position. Some conditions should be categorized in two and sometimes three of the categories. When planning a session, you won't know the absolute adjustments until you meet the client. At this point, they are possible adjustments.

1. Type of cancer and location: *Left BR CA, stage 3, estrogen/progesterone receptor positive*

2. Date of diagnosis: *Feb. 20, 2014 (8 months ago)*

3. Presently in treatment?   No   (Yes)

If yes, what type? *Radiation (5 treatments remaining)*

If no, when did treatment end?

4. TREATMENT REVIEW:

				Year
Surgery:	No (Yes)	Describe	*Mastectomy with 12 lymph nodes removed.*	2014
			7 months since surgery.	
Radiation:	No (Yes)	Area	*Left chest, including axilla, clavicle to bottom*	2014
			of breast. Completed 28 of 33 treatments.	
Chemo:	No (Yes)	Rounds	*6 rounds over 18 weeks.*	2014
			Finished 6 weeks ago.	

5. REVIEW of SIDE EFFECTS and HEALTH CONSIDERATIONS

Pressure Adjustments:

Systemic pressure adjustments:
Fatigue
Zoloft (anti-depressant)

What overall pressure would you use for this client? *2*
List the reasons: *Fatigue, presently in treatment, months of treatment prior to present one.*

Continued on page 2

Appendix 5c *Client A: Massage Session Planning* Worksheet 2 of 2

Local pressure adjustments:

Risk of lymphedema—L upper quadrant
Surgical and radiation site—L chest, shoulder
CIPN—toes
Joints affected by chemo pain

Site Restrictions:

Areas to be mindful of:

Left chest and shoulder due to surgery and radiation
Protects neck and left shoulder
Numbness/prickling under left arm and axilla
Toes due to CIPN
Joint pain

Are there areas on which you *might* use less pressure from the overall pressure listed earlier?
List those areas below:

Left upper quadrant (risk of lymphedema)
Surgical and radiation site
Neck and left shoulder
Toes (CIPN)
Joints affected by chemo pain

Positioning Adjustments:

She may not want to lie prone due to radiation and mastectomy
Suggest right side-lying

6. What further clarifications would you want from this client?

How would you rate your energy compared to pre-diagnosis?
I would ask her to show me the range of movement in her neck and shoulder.
I would also want her to show me the exact field of treatment of the radiation.
What side effects are the medications causing?
What information has your health care team given you about lymphedema? Or what have you
learned on your own?
In which toes or parts of your toes do you experience peripheral neuropathy.?

Appendix 6 *Body Map* Worksheet

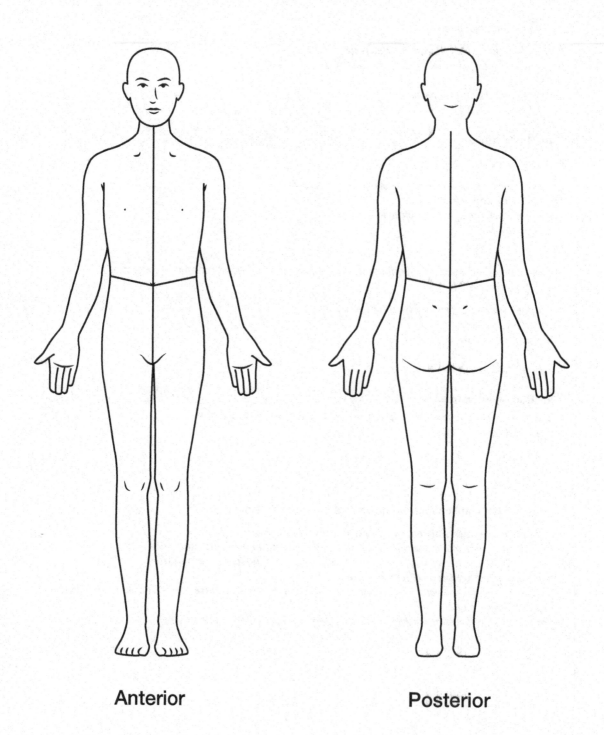

Anterior   **Posterior**

Appendix 7 *Reflection Space* Worksheet

Reflection Space

Findhorn Press recommends…

Medicine Hands, 3rd Edition

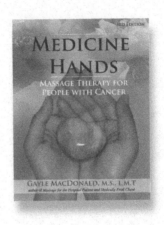

Other massage books

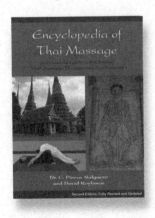

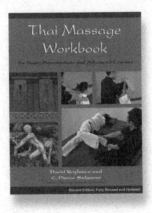

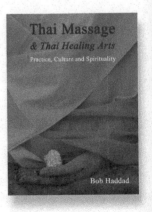

FINDHORN PRESS

Life-Changing Books

Consult our catalogue online
(with secure order facility) on
www.findhornpress.com

For information on the Findhorn Foundation:
www.findhorn.org